RA 972.7
A38
1974

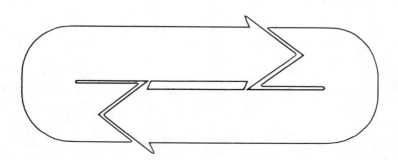

The Auxiliary:
New Concepts, New Directions

American Hospital Association
840 North Lake Shore Drive
Chicago, Illinois 60611

312972

Library of Congress Cataloging in Publication Data
American Hospital Association.
    The auxiliary: new concepts, new directions.
    Bibliography: p.
    Includes index.
    1. Volunteer workers in hospitals. I. Title.
[DNLM: 1. Hospital volunteers. WX150 A511a]
RA972.7.A43   1974a   658.3'04   74-22174
ISBN 0-87258-160-8

M93
13.5M-12/74-4008   **1M-12/81-7924**

AHA Catalog no. 019110
© 1974 by the
American Hospital Association
840 North Lake Shore Drive
Chicago, Illinois 60611
Printed in the U.S.A.

Contents

Preface

This manual has been written to provide auxilians, and the institutions they serve, with a new perspective on the auxiliary's role and responsibilities. It replaces the out-of-date *Patterns and Principles for Hospital Auxiliaries*, published by the American Hospital Association in 1957.

In helping their institutions to better meet community health needs, auxiliaries must from time to time examine their own concepts of service to institution and community. In doing so, they may discover that it is necessary to redefine their purpose and objectives, revise their organizational structure and methods of operation, and expand their concepts of service to new dimensions appropriate to the changing demands of today and tomorrow.

Auxiliaries are individual organizations, each with its particular needs, problems, and modes of functioning. Each should therefore view the new concepts and directions set forth in this book not as a rigid set of rules but as guidelines to be studied and utilized in the context of the auxiliary's own situation.

The type of ownership of the institution served by the auxiliary is one factor that must be taken into consideration in utilizing these guidelines. For example, auxiliaries serving investor-owned or government hospitals may find that not all the information is applicable to their organizations without modification and, in particular, should seek the advice of their institutions' attorneys on such subjects as legal organization, utilization of auxilians in inservice volunteer programs, and financial structure.

In the shaping of the manual, a great many persons have contributed their philosophies, ideas, and viewpoints. The Association is grateful for their interest and unstinting assistance, and for the skill with which Sandra E. Fink, the book's principal author, has presented the material.

chapter 1
The Role of the Auxiliary

When some form of national health insurance seems
imminent, when entire new systems for the delivery of health
care are being designed, when citizen groups,
eager to exercise "patient power," are organizing all over
the country — what are auxiliaries doing to determine
the new obligations and responsibilities to hospital and community
which the health care upheaval has presented to them?
What opportunities for service lie ahead of us if we can develop
our organizations into groups responsive to the
new needs of our times?

Mrs. Newton Millham,
former chairman,
Committee on Volunteers,
American Hospital Association

New Concepts, New Needs

Health care institutions are in the process of change,
evolving from inner-directed and self-contained units into entities
that encompass total health care for their communities.

Responding to revolutionary advances in medical science and
to consumer demands for more comprehensive and accessible
health care, the delivery system for health services is expanding
to meet newly emerging needs. The hospital — once the primary
source of institutional health care — is becoming the central
entity in a continuum of institutions, with ambulatory care
assuming an increasingly important role in the provision of

health services. Within this comprehensive system, coordinated services, including acute care, extended and home care, rehabilitation, and programs for community health education and disease prevention, are offered through a variety of facilities.

As noted in the American Hospital Association's *Statement on Optimum Health Services,* the move is toward a "coordinated community and/or regional system that incorporates the full spectrum of health services and provides for coordination of care from the time of the patient's primary contact with the system through the community hospital to the university hospital and/or medical center and other health agencies. Each [health care institution] should provide the portion of the total spectrum of health services that is feasible in terms of the type of community it serves and the overall pattern of health facilities of the region in which it exists" (ref. 9).

Simply stated, the health care institution cannot stand aloof from the community; it is *of* the community. In order to provide optimum health care services, the institution must be responsive to the community's health needs and must seek out the assistance of individuals throughout the community in planning ways to meet these needs.

As the role of the health care institution changes, the role of the auxiliary must be modified, for the auxiliary's first responsibility always has been to serve its institution. From the moment of the auxiliary's inception, and as long as it exists, there is a binding relationship between the two entities — rooted in the auxiliary's primary purpose and in its acceptance by the institution as an integral part of the institutional family. As the auxiliary comes to identify the institution's goals as its own and to generate programs of service that are responsive to its institution's changing needs, it becomes an effective device for accomplishing mutual objectives. Therefore, to truly represent its institution in the most contemporary sense, the auxiliary must join it in promoting the health and welfare of those in the community — not only of those within the four walls of the physical facility.

The Challenge: Broader Dimensions of Service

As the auxiliary seeks to shape a vital new role appropriate to the 1970s and 1980s, it will discover that there are no traditional formulas to follow. The movement is toward unexplored concepts of service and untried areas of activity. It is the auxiliary's responsibility to anticipate the changing health care requirements of its institution and community and to develop new directions of activity. The auxiliary and the administration should start by envisioning the auxiliary in all the following roles:

Pioneer of Fresh Approaches to Improve Health Care Delivery

The role of the auxiliary as innovator reflects the broader concept of service that is emerging. Acting with the support and the approval of its institution's chief executive, the auxiliary should devise plans of action to help establish new and needed programs, such as a neighborhood health clinic. In other instances, the auxiliary may wisely conclude that it is not necessary to initiate a service in order to perform one. Being innovative, it should make better use of existing health care resources by joining forces with other agencies to promote the voluntary donation of blood, for example, or by working with neighborhood schools to enrich health education.

Community Relations Agent

In the past, the auxiliary was primarily concerned with efforts to make the community better understand and appreciate the institution. Now, it is also imperative that the auxiliary help its institution to more fully comprehend and appreciate the community — its sociological structure, its health care needs, its attitudes toward available services, and its resources. A diversified auxiliary membership, truly representative and reflective of the community, is an excellent source for such information. (See page 14 of this manual.)

At the same time, the auxiliary retains the traditional responsibility for helping the community learn about the services its institution offers, the financial needs of the institution and ways in which they can best be met, the policies of the institution and the reasons they are necessary, and the serious operating problems faced every day by the institution. Of particular importance is promoting community understanding of the institution's cost structure and its validity. Public support and interest can be successfully created when this vital information is fully and skillfully presented throughout the year — not only during fundraising campaigns.

Champion of Issues

Most auxilians correctly perceive that the role of champion of issues historically has been reserved for the hospital administration, the board of trustees, and the medical staff. However, history in no way should restrain the auxiliary from participating in this function and utilizing its influence — *provided that* its role is clearly understood and accepted by all parties involved and affected. Participation as champion of issues is both a logical extension of the capabilities of auxilians and a largely untapped resource for effecting change that strengthens and improves the health care delivery system.

In order to participate intelligently, auxiliary members should be prepared to present to the administration for approval an organized plan of action, aimed at achieving specific, mutually acceptable objectives. In developing its recommendations, the auxiliary should first make a careful study of the urgent health care issues affecting the institution and the community. Because they are myriad, the auxiliary must be prepared to decide which issues most urgently and logically deserve its support.

For instance, should there be combined action by the institution, the schools, and the community on such pressing matters as mental illness, health education, and environmental protection? Would involvement by auxilians in legislative activities that relate to the health care field at both state and national levels be productive in resolving the identified urgent issues?

The auxiliary also can act as spokesman on needs arising from the areas it is closest to, such as the importance of the psychological aspects of health care. How do the poor, the old, and members of minority groups fare in getting their share of services? What kind of help is offered the non-English-speaking patient? Is attention given to the human needs of the alcoholic when he is undergoing treatment? Are counseling services available to offer solutions to widespread social problems, such as drug addiction and venereal disease? What kind of emotional support is provided for the terminally ill and their families?

In making its voice heard through its institution, the auxiliary can become a positive force in helping to meet such needs.

The Continuing Responsibility: Traditional Programs

While the auxiliary is reaching out in new directions, it should continue its work in traditional programs. Certain traditional auxiliary services that the institution wants and needs will continue to make demands on the auxiliary's energy and resourcefulness. The auxiliary should be willing to periodically reevaluate which of these basic programs are serving an important purpose and which have outlived their usefulness. When such programs are retained, the auxiliary should seek ways to improve them.

Among the most common traditional programs are the following:

Supporting Inservice Volunteer Program

The auxiliary can be of great assistance not only in recruiting volunteers for the institution's inservice program but also in suggesting useful ways to utilize their time and talents. However, the auxiliary should not interpret its supportive role as a supervisory one unless that responsibility has been specifically assigned to the auxiliary by the hospital's chief executive officer. The auxiliary should also guard against being equated solely with the inservice program or being viewed merely as an appendage of the volunteer services department.

Fund Raising

Fund raising by the auxiliary is important to help meet the institution's capital needs and to support institutional and community health programs for which outside financing may be unavailable. Ways and means of fund raising should be carefully considered, however, to ensure that this activity reflects favorably on the image of the auxiliary and the institution. (See Chapter 7.)

Opportunities and Expectations

Throughout the years, auxiliaries have responded to the needs of their institutions and in their response have demonstrated their great value. Today new needs have opened wider the doors of opportunity for service. Because auxiliaries have proved their flexibility and their diverse capabilities so convincingly in the past, much more is expected of them now.

chapter 2
The Auxiliary's Accountabilities and Relationships

If hospitals are to do the job the public is expecting
of them in the years ahead, they must make greater use of
all community resources. Auxilians have untapped potential as
community resources, but that potential will remain
unrealized unless administrators take a new look at and
adopt a new attitude toward their own auxilians.

Robert M. Sigmond,
executive vice president,
Albert Einstein Medical Center, Philadelphia

An auxiliary is founded by persons from the community who
agree to work together to assist a health care institution in promoting the health and welfare of the community. By formalizing
their agreement and establishing an organization, the founders
create a responsible entity with a legal personality.

However, this new entity can function as an auxiliary only by
authorization of the institution's governing board. Hence, the
governing board, in effect, confers on an auxiliary:

- Identification with the institution.
- The right to manage its own internal affairs.
- The responsibility for helping to further the institution's
  purpose and goals through activities that are both appropriate to and within the capabilities of a community volunteer organization.

At the same time, the governing board retains the right, exercised through its chief executive officer, to review and approve
activities and programs undertaken by the auxiliary for the insti-

tution. Therefore, as an inherent part of its delegated responsibility, the auxiliary automatically assumes the obligation to be accountable to its institution for the exercise of the authority entrusted to it.

The Administration and the Auxiliary

One way in which this accountability is expressed is through the development of a strong relationship between the auxiliary and the administration, founded on close communication and mutual respect.

The president of the auxiliary plays the role of chief liaison officer between the auxiliary and the institution's administration. By her attitudes and actions she, in large measure, determines the kind of relationship that will exist between auxiliary and institution.*

Regularly scheduled conferences between the auxiliary president and the chief executive, or his representative, go far toward establishing the best possible relationship. Such conferences offer opportunities for a discussion of plans being considered by the institution and the auxiliary and for a review of projects under way. Because they are regularly scheduled, they also have a preventive value, confronting potential problems before they become major concerns and averting crisis situations.

If the auxiliary president is handling her role as chief liaison officer effectively, it is rarely necessary for the chief executive to attend all meetings of the auxiliary's board or general membership. In any event, the auxiliary president should regularly send the meeting agenda and minutes to him, being careful to indicate any items demanding his attention. In this way, the auxiliary president keeps the chief executive informed about auxiliary activities and alert to the times when his advice and counsel are needed or his attendance may be indicated.

This approach to a vitally important relationship indicates an attitude of healthy independence on the auxiliary's part. Many auxiliaries have a tendency to seek approval from their chief executive on even the smallest decision. This can create problems for both the chief executive and the auxiliary — for him, in terms

---

*The use of *she* and *her* in referring to auxilians, and of *he* and *him* in referring to chief executive officers, is an editorial convenience, not an implication that every auxilian is female and every chief executive officer male.

of expenditure of time, and for the auxiliary, in terms of developing strong leadership. It is therefore the quality of the chief executive's involvement, rather than the quantity of time he contributes, that is significant.

When the auxiliary president and the chief executive work as a team, the auxiliary becomes more knowledgeable about the institution and more aware of its services and needs. Equally important, the administration comes to view the auxiliary in two important lights:

- As a trusted member of the institution's team, to be apprised of current issues facing the institution and the health care field and involved in discussion of the institution's long-range plans.
- As a community resource, to be consulted in determining community attitudes and capable of initiating and carrying out community-oriented projects.

The Chief Executive and the Auxiliary President

In light of the new expectations of auxiliaries in the 1970s and 1980s, the chief executive and the auxiliary president must probe many mutual areas of concern. The following questions may serve as a basis for discussion:

- How can the present role of the auxiliary be enriched and expanded, thus extending the range of current activities?
- What roles will the auxiliary play in the future, in terms of the institution and the community, particularly regarding the delivery of better health care?
- In what ways can the auxiliary be helped to develop realistic expectations of the administration, and the administration to develop realistic expectations of the auxiliary?
- How can communication between the chief executive and the auxiliary president be made more satisfactory to both and a freer exchange of ideas promoted?
- What provisions can be made to ensure that the chief executive shares the institution's problems with the auxiliary president and involves the auxiliary more closely in long-range planning for the institution?
- How can more open and direct communication be encouraged between the institution and the community? What are the community's feelings about the work of the auxiliary and

its effectiveness in helping its institution meet community health care problems? How does the community regard the institution itself in terms of responsiveness to the community's health needs?

- How can the auxiliary improve its relationship with other members of the institution's family, such as medical staff, trustees, department heads, and employees?

The Governing Board and the Auxiliary

Whether the president should represent the auxiliary on the institution's governing board is a question that concerns many auxiliaries. There are two points of view. One school holds that because the president represents an important organization that is part and parcel of the total institutional structure, she should be an ex officio member of the governing board. The other insists that governing board members should be chosen for their qualifications, not for the organizations or groups they represent. According to this latter school, an auxilian might well sit on the governing board — not, however, because of her auxiliary connections, but because, as an individual, she can contribute to the board's deliberations. The American Hospital Association belongs to the second school of thought, but it respects the decision of those governing boards that wish to invite auxiliary representation.

Although there are two possible approaches to this particular question, there is only one feasible attitude for an auxiliary to take: it must leave the decision to the governing board and be willing to abide by that decision, whatever it may be. There is also only one attitude that an auxiliary representative on the governing board should assume: she must remember that she is functioning in two capacities, and therefore she should never, in her relationship with the administration, presume on her board connection. Despite a president's presence on the governing board, the auxiliary continues to operate under the guidance of the administration.

Of much greater import than whether the auxiliary president serves on the institution's board is the extent to which the auxiliary is integrated into board activities. This integrative process can best be accomplished when auxilians are given the opportunity to serve on various board committees, such as long-range planning, public or community relations, and fund raising. To assist this process, the auxiliary should suggest the names of its members (not necessarily officers) who are particularly well qualified to serve on board committees.

Integration is further enhanced if the board views auxilians as important resource persons, oriented to issues and capable of helping the institution resolve major problems.

The ultimate objective, of course, is more intensive auxiliary participation in the institution's affairs — an object of far greater importance than mere token auxiliary representation on the board.

The Community and the Auxiliary

One of the strengths of the auxiliary lies in the fact that it is an organization *of* the community, dedicated to serving a community institution. As such, it should make connections with other local groups in order to initiate and develop solid community relationships. Beyond this, however, the auxiliary should utilize the expertise of those organizations that touch upon the auxiliary's interests in some way. The auxiliary can seek assistance in developing programs for its institution and, when appropriate, can invite the participation of these groups in joining projects for the community.

An auxiliary wishing to become involved in a *blood procurement program* for its institution, for example, can either participate in an existing program at the hospital or contact its local Red Cross chapter for assistance in establishing and conducting this type of endeavor if the hospital needs and wants it (see ref. 2).

Another possibility would be an information program to encourage a total blood donation commitment by a community. This program could utilize both auxilians and volunteers who can assist the local Red Cross chapter in disseminating facts about blood needs. The auxiliary could also assume responsibility for developing a communitywide blood procurement program. It is desirable that the promotion of programs with outside agencies, and the development of cooperative information programs, be conducted in conjunction with the institution's public relations-community relations department, if it exists, in order to ensure proper coordination of effort.

Organized activity on behalf of health care legislation is another area in which the contemporary auxiliary will want to become involved (see ref. 5). The hospital association in each state is the appropriate entry point for auxilians wishing to gain information and guidelines on participation in legislative action programs. Another resource is the American Hospital Association's Washington office, which coordinates the Association's legislative activities and depends upon assistance from the state hospital associations in order to influence the outcome of federal health care legislation. The auxiliary can also consult with the chief executive of its institution for help in this activity. Outside of the health care field, other organizations can be valuable resources for gathering information. An example is the local office of the League of Women Voters, which can supply facts on the procedures and approaches for involvement in legislative action programs.

As described in Chapter 7, "Fund Raising," there are a number of possibilities for joint projects and programs with other community organizations and agencies. The pooling of funds, organizational skills, and manpower can frequently launch a program more effectively and efficiently than the efforts of the auxiliary alone. Local groups such as mental health associations, visiting nurse organizations, private social welfare agencies, and other auxiliaries are potential sources for information on the community's health care and health education needs and for operational assistance in the development and implementation of such programs.

The modern auxiliary recognizes that it can be a giver — to other community organizations — as well as a receiver of their resources in personnel, know-how, and community contacts. The auxiliary, too, has great resources that can be valuable to others. It has personnel with special talents and knowledge; it has organizational structure and sometimes funds to assist community groups in accomplishing missions that are compatible with the auxiliary's own. It has a responsibility to the community to share its resources when sharing can serve to enhance its own goals and those of its institution.

chapter 3
Membership and Leadership

When the best leader's work is done the people say,
"We did it ourselves!"

Lao-tzu,
Chinese philosopher,
Circa 604-531 B.C.

Members are the substance of the auxiliary. As individuals working together for a common purpose, they sustain their organization through their collective action and, in the process, learn what each of them is capable of accomplishing. It is through this demonstration of an individual's contributions to the overall development of the auxiliary that the first suggestions of leadership potential are provided.

Leadership evolves from membership through a process of growth, nurtured by the ability of the auxiliary's leaders to maintain a climate that encourages the development of leadership qualities. It is the force that transforms the energies, resources, and commitments of the individual members into effective service for the ongoing benefit of the institution and, at the same time, propels to the forefront those capable of assuming leadership responsibilities in the future. The evolution of membership into leadership is a continuing process that perpetually renews itself. As successive generations of leaders are drawn from the ranks, they, in turn, help to develop the leadership abilities of *their* successors, and so it goes.

Open Membership

No provision in the auxiliary's bylaws is more important — or more revealing of the auxiliary's understanding of its role and responsibilities — than the provision that sets forth its membership policy.

By pursuing a policy of open membership, the auxiliary clearly recognizes that, as a community organization serving a community institution, its strength lies in the diversity and representative nature of its membership. Its capacity to provide service depends on its ability to draw upon many different kinds of talents. Its effectiveness as a link in the institution's communication chain depends on whether its members are truly representative of all sectors of the community it serves. By limiting auxiliary membership to adults within the community, the auxiliary underscores the importance of experience and mature judgment to the realization of its goals. With the exception of this one limitation, auxiliary membership should be open.

A policy of open membership must, of course, be true in spirit as well as in fact. In order to accomplish this, an auxiliary should examine its own inner attitudes to determine whether it truly wants a representative membership and what it has to offer that will attract members from all strata of the community. If the auxiliary's programs and activities are meaningful and demonstrate real concern for the community's health care needs, this will eventually become apparent to those the auxiliary needs to reach. As community trust grows, so will membership.

The following questions can help auxilians ascertain whether their auxiliary has, inadvertently, been limiting membership:

- Has the auxiliary made an active effort to recruit auxilians from every area of the community?
- Are men welcome in the organization and given the opportunity to play a vital role?
- Are meeting times scheduled so that those employed full time can attend?
- Is the auxiliary placing undue emphasis on the kinds of activities — formal dinners, pool parties, fashion shows — that label it as an exclusive club?
- Is the orientation program for new members designed to make many different kinds of people feel comfortable with

the group and help them find a useful place in the organization?

Recruitment

The recruitment process offers the auxiliary an unparalleled opportunity to become a true community volunteer organization. It is a starting point in establishing strong ties to the community and in initiating communication between the consumers of health care services and the provider institution. In recruiting potential auxilians, certain principles should apply if the process is to produce a corps of dedicated and productive individuals.

Principles

Recruitment should be conducted from among all racial, religious, ethnic, economic, educational, and age groups in the community — a representative cross section. This means enlisting senior citizens and young adults to balance the middle-aged component within the auxiliary, appealing to men to view themselves as potential auxiliary members, and making representatives of minority groups aware of the need for their services. The primary consideration in creating a diverse membership is, of course, the actual composition of the community, which may or may not be structured to provide auxilians from all these groups.

The auxiliary should offer enough variety in its programs and projects to appeal to a wide assortment of individuals. To attract meaningful participation, the auxiliary should provide activities that are meaningful to the institution and the community. In seeking out younger persons as members, for example, the auxiliary competes with other community organizations that are also recruiting — a cogent reason for offering the kinds of programs that will attract the interest of younger volunteers within the broader appeal to all kinds of individuals.

When the auxiliary conducts projects that demand unusual numbers of volunteers or persons with specialized talents and the need is urgent, participants can be derived from the community on a project basis, without auxiliary membership being required for involvement.

Knowledge of the community's structure, in terms of its leadership and organizations, and establishment of working relationships with these entities are essential elements in the recruitment process as well as in the auxiliary's overall functioning. Enlisting the help of the community in recruiting members, therefore, becomes a natural outgrowth of this interrelationship. This cooperation is particularly relevant for auxiliaries serving institutions without community relations departments, which normally would perform this service on the auxiliary's behalf.

Group membership, described later in this chapter, is another excellent means of involving the community in the auxiliary's work and of stimulating individuals to join. It is also a useful device for achieving diversification.

The effectiveness of recruitment efforts should be evaluated periodically. If an auxiliary is not drawing the number of members it needs or the type of community representation it desires, the problem could reside either in the image the auxiliary projects or in its methods of recruitment; for reaching the appropriate persons becomes a questionable accomplishment if, once reached, they fail to respond. If an auxiliary has been characterized by snob values, exclusivity, uninteresting and unimaginative programs and projects, or a nonresponsive attitude to community needs, it will have difficulty in motivating others to join.

A dynamic auxiliary — contemporary in its viewpoint, responsive to needs, and flexible enough to accommodate change — will attract the number and kinds of persons it needs.

Techniques

Two major areas should be explored and used in recruiting volunteers: other community organizations and the local media.

Volunteer action centers and volunteer bureaus are among the community organizations that can provide help in recruitment procedures. In many communities, these agencies serve as referral centers for volunteer placement, matching available volunteers with organizations that need them most.

It could also be advantageous for the auxiliary to contact local United Way affiliates and inform them that it is conducting a recruitment drive for volunteers. These organizations, which are known variously as the Crusade of Mercy, Community Fund,

United Community Services, or Community Council, are often tuned into volunteer availabilities within their given communities.

If there are no voluntary action centers or volunteer bureaus in the community, the auxiliary could conduct a joint recruitment, interviewing, and placement effort with other local health care institutions and/or community organizations, such as the Red Cross or the Visiting Nurse Association. A central clearinghouse could be established to operate the program and to provide all participating agencies and institutions with information on available volunteers. This clearinghouse would then become the local contact point for volunteers.

To disseminate information about volunteer recruitment efforts, the auxiliary should become knowledgeable about local media and acquainted with the key personnel on newspaper staffs and at radio and television stations. Because volunteering for a health care institution is obviously a public service, the auxiliary frequently can obtain free radio and television time for interviews and public service spot announcements. Newspaper space often is available for public service editorials and news items promoting the recruitment drive. In addition, the auxiliary may wish to purchase advertising.

The auxiliary should work with the public relations-community relations department of its institution to develop the proper channels of communication with the media and community organizations. If such a department does not exist, the auxiliary should work directly with the administration in these areas.

A Formal Application

Membership that is open but without commitment is meaningless. It becomes meaningful when the established policy requires a formal application from the prospective member, pledging loyalty to the auxiliary and to the institution it serves, and an acceptance of that pledge by the auxiliary. The giving and the accepting of such a pledge attest that both the member and the organization recognize that each has an obligation to the other. The sample application form shown on page 18 illustrates the type of document suggested.

Dues

Dues are another reflection of membership policy. If they are nominal and offer no serious bar to membership, they

APPLICATION FOR AUXILIARY MEMBERSHIP

_____
(Name of auxiliary)

I hereby make application for membership in the auxiliary
for the year ending_____
(Month)   (Year)

I agree to uphold the purpose and policies of the auxiliary
and the institution that it serves. I understand that my
membership is renewed upon payment of annual dues.
Payment of $_____for the current year is enclosed.

SIGNATURE _____

NAME (print) _____

ADDRESS_____

_____

TELEPHONE NO. _____

Date_____

underscore the auxiliary's dedication to a membership that is
open to all adults interested in the institution and willing to
uphold the auxiliary's purpose. On the other hand, dues should
be realistic, for they provide the auxiliary's operating budget.
It is suggested that annual dues range from $1 to $10.

No auxiliary can operate without income to cover its administrative expenses and thus make possible its total program. It is
both logical and appropriate that the organization should look to
its members to provide this operating income as one indication
of their personal commitment. (See Appendix A, model bylaws,
Article IV, Dues.)

The collection of delinquent dues can be a sensitive area. Unless
a definite and firm position is taken on the time limit for the
payment of dues, the auxiliary can be left in limbo for an inordi-

nate period regarding not only the receipt of dues but also the individual's desire to continue membership. Rather than prolonging the agony, the auxiliary should establish a period of three months from the start of the fiscal year as an adequate amount of time in which to pay dues. If the dues are still delinquent after this period has passed, the member should be dropped.

Types of Membership

Individual Membership

Individual membership encompasses the following types:

Regular. It is recommended that there be no differentiation into active, inactive, sustaining, or associate memberships. Even the added income from the higher dues often paid by those members who are classified (sometimes only temporarily) as inactive or sustaining is rarely sufficient to justify the additional record keeping. In summation, all members are members — but some are more active than others!

Honorary. This form of membership offers the auxiliary a most acceptable means of recognizing outstanding service performed by an individual (not necessarily an auxilian). It also provides an opportunity for the auxiliary to interact with the community in the selection of recipients. This membership is distinct from regular membership and does not, of itself, grant to the honorary member the right to vote or hold office. In order to exercise these privileges, the honorary member must also meet the requirements for being a member in good standing, including payment of dues.

Life. Life memberships, which are traditional in many auxiliaries, are usually used as a fund-raising device. Within this membership classification, individuals are given the opportunity to make a major financial contribution (usually not less than $100) and, presumably, a lifelong commitment to the auxiliary. The possibility may be overlooked that an individual who joins the auxiliary on this basis could become a personal liability. It could be difficult or even impossible to legitimately insist on the member's resignation. The only protection for the auxiliary that wishes to maintain a life membership category is to choose such members with great discretion. However, it is recommended that the auxiliary consider omitting life memberships entirely.

Group Membership

A group membership is held in the name of another organization in the community, as a means of indicating its support for and interest in the institution and the health care field. If this form of membership seems advisable to the auxiliary and acceptable to the institution, it should be provided for in the bylaws and should require the same commitment from the group member as that asked of the individual member. In other words, that section of the bylaws authorizing group membership should state:

Membership in the auxiliary shall also be open to any organization made up of adults that is interested in (name of health care institution) and willing to uphold the purpose of the auxiliary. Membership shall become effective when the signed application for membership is approved by majority vote of the board of directors present at a regular meeting and when the initial dues are paid.

Other sections in the bylaws should specify: the amount of annual dues to be paid by the group member (these should be nominal, usually $5 or $10) ; the number of representatives of the group who may formally represent the organization; whether the group member is entitled to one vote or a number of votes equal to the number of its formal representatives; whether any individual member of the group has a right to hold elective office in the auxiliary or sit on the board of directors; and the responsibility of the group member for providing to the auxiliary, at the beginning of each fiscal year, the names of those persons who will represent the group. The bylaws also should provide for the possibility of the group member's resignation and should permit the auxiliary's board of directors, at its discretion, to refuse to renew a group membership.

Many an auxiliary has found that providing group memberships is an excellent method for involving the total community in activities that benefit its hospital or other health care facility. However, the decision to establish this form of membership should be made with the realization that other organizations have their own primary purposes and concerns, and they therefore may be unable to make a firm commitment to the auxiliary's goals.

Liaison Membership

The bylaws can also authorize liaison membership, which permits another organization in the community to send a representative to auxiliary meetings in order to report on the auxiliary's activities. Groups holding liaison membership do not pay dues and are not allowed to vote. By offering this type of membership, the auxiliary opens up more channels of communication within the community and takes a positive step toward ending fragmentation and duplication of services.

Obligations to Members

The vitality of an auxiliary depends on how successfully its leadership infuses membership with the desire to participate. Leadership can stimulate this desire to participate in the following ways:

Uncover Needs and Talents

Each member is an individual with different human needs to be satisfied and assorted skills, interests, and experience to offer. The auxiliary has a continuing obligation to try to understand and meet each person's special needs and to utilize to the fullest her particular abilities.

Offer Opportunities for Participation

Having ascertained needs and talents, the auxiliary must offer its members meaningful participation in its activities, for commitment grows as the individual becomes involved in the larger purpose of the organization. Through participation the individual comes to understand the significance of membership: accepting a job that is serious and contributory, assuming responsibility for the job assigned, and fulfilling high standards of performance.

Offer a Voice in Decision Making

Participation cannot be truly meaningful if the general membership is expected only to carry out projects decided upon by the auxiliary's board, without ever being consulted in the planning stages. The board must constantly weigh efficiency — the need to get the job done — against the long-range benefits of total membership participation in making major decisions.

The wise board will take the long-range point of view, seeking membership approval and consequent support for proposals that will require additional or extraordinary effort in membership service, time, or money. As an added benefit, the auxiliary that involves its membership in making as well as executing plans is, at the same time, contributing to member education.

Provide Tools

In evaluating how well its members are equipped for their responsibilities, the auxiliary should ask itself the following questions: Does every member have a copy of the current by-laws? Do all officers and committee chairmen have an up-to-date copy of administrative policies and procedures, and is the membership aware of changes as they are being made? Do the chairmen and all members of all committees have a written statement of the committee's purpose, functions, responsibilities, and relationships?

Does every member have ready access to reference material published by national and state hospital associations as well as other publications that apply to activities of the auxiliary? Is every member aware that such references exist? Is every member also aware of the services and consultation available from state and national associations?

Does member education include orientation sessions for new members, workshops for more experienced members, and informative meeting programs? Does the auxiliary make it possible for some members to attend appropriate educational meetings sponsored by district, state, regional, and national hospital associations, and local health and welfare agencies? These educational opportunities continually contribute to the growth of the individual and augment her knowledge of the institution and the health care field.

Provide Opportunity for Advancement

Opportunity for advancement by itself is not enough; there also must be its corollary — training for increased responsibility. Conversely, training without opportunity is equally hazardous, for the well-trained member with no place to go within the organization is apt to become another statistic in the auxiliary dropout rate. Not all members may want to assume increased responsibility, but the opportunity and the encouragment offered by training should be available.

Opportunity exists when the bylaws limit the terms of officers and committee chairmen and the number of consecutive years any one person may serve on the board of directors. Encouragement is offered when the bylaws provide for more than one vice president, one or more assistant secretaries and treasurers, and a vice chairman as well as a chairman for each standing committee. Realization of both opportunity and encouragement, however, rests with a functioning nominating committee, responsible membership relations and membership education committees, and an organization dedicated to the proposition that both leadership and progress are products of the auxiliary's concern for membership.

Provide Recognition

The auxiliary's final obligation to its members is to provide recognition for service. However, "too often, recognition is equated with awards, when, in fact, other types of recognition carry greater personal significance. To the individual, one of the most satisfying kinds of recognition is the knowledge that his efforts alone assure the completion of certain tasks. . . . To stress this intangible recognition of volunteer service in no way negates the value or use of tangible awards under the right circumstances. Instead, it places the emphasis where it belongs — on service. In the final analysis, the type and amount of recognition given the volunteer depend on the individual health care institution and the volunteer service organization" (ref. 10).

The forms of recognition to be discussed here are intangible (as contrasted to the tangible and more traditional pin, plaque, or certificate) and emanate from the auxiliary, the institution, and the community.

Beginning with the auxiliary, election to an office or appointment to the chairmanship of a committee is recognition of an individual's leadership potential or affirmation of excellent performance in a previous leadership position. Sending representatives of the general membership to educational institutes or to local, state, and national meetings pertaining to health care is another form of recognition.

Recognition is also provided when auxiliary representation on the committees or boards of community groups is directly sought by these outside organizations. When the institution is requested to supply a representative to a community group and suggests that an auxilian fill this position, this, too, indicates that the auxiliary is valued.

Via publicity placed with the local media, the auxiliary can work to promote the accomplishments of individual members, the auxiliary as a group, and the auxiliary in cooperation with other community organizations. This should be done, of course, in conjunction with the institution's public relations-community relations department. Such publicity can result in community recognition of the auxiliary's services, as described later in this section. The auxiliary's newsletter and annual report offer an opportunity for periodic recognition of individual effort as well as acknowledgment of group achievement.

Recognition from the institution can be expressed by an invitation to an auxilian to serve on the hospital's governing board. A recognition day held at the institution is another possibility, with friends, family, and the community invited to an informal open house at which both auxilians and volunteers are honored. Photographs of those being cited, with descriptive captions, could be displayed in some central location during the event. This use of auxilians' and volunteers' photographs can also be employed as a year-round form of recognition within the institution, with photos displayed on staff bulletin boards or in other highly visible locations. National Hospital Week could be an appropriate time to schedule a recognition day, with accompanying publicity.

In addition, the institution's newsletter to the community or the house publication for professional staff and employees can devote a special issue to honoring the auxiliary and the department of volunteer services. A special newsletter for patients could also be utilized for this purpose.

Community recognition can be a most satisfying experience for the auxiliary, whether individual auxilians are singled out for performance or the group is cited for achievement. Should community organizations decide to provide this recognition via special awards, this is yet another indication that the auxiliary's accomplishments are appreciated.

For a detailed discussion of this subject, see the American Hospital Association publication *Volunteer Recognition and Identification* (ref. 10).

Recognize Less Active Members

Despite the auxiliary's best efforts to fulfill its obligations to all its members, there may be a few individuals who are unable or unwilling to contribute more than their loyalty and their dues. Such a situation should not cause the auxiliary undue concern, once it has been established that certain members honestly wish to make no greater commitment. Conversely, these same members deserve more from the auxiliary than an annual statement of dues. They should be kept well informed of auxiliary projects and problems in anticipation that eventually they, too, will become more active members.

The Nature of Leadership

The kind of leadership an auxiliary wants and needs rarely develops spontaneously and should not be left to chance. Simply stated, leadership is behavior that influences others to act. Consequently, it is possible for an organization to:

- Assess an individual's potential for leadership and provide opportunity to develop it.
- Predict the kind of leadership, or influence, an individual will exercise by observing her patterns of behavior, and then choose leadership that generally reflects the organization's goals.
- Determine, by its choice of leadership, the manner in which it will attain its purpose, for organizations tend to assume the character and personality of their leaders.

These seeming abstractions have very real meaning for the auxiliary. First, it should be assumed that every member has a capacity for leadership. Acting on this assumption, the auxiliary will constantly search the total membership for potential leaders, overlooking no one and often discovering what might otherwise remain hidden talent. Further, it will provide opportunities to develop leadership capacity to all who indicate both potential and interest.

Second, the auxiliary demonstrates its clarity of purpose by the kind of leadership it selects. Given the behavioral nature of leadership, the organization will determine its own course of action by choosing those whose ideas of the auxiliary's basic purpose and responsibilities generally correspond to the group's own understanding of these principles.

Finally, the way in which an organization pursues its goals is also determined by its choice of leadership, because a group reflects the character and personality of its leader in its method of approach and operation. For example, the organization that accepts the fact that change and innovation are essential will select as its leader a bold, dynamic personality capable of initiating new directions. Conversely, a more conservative group will choose a leader who accords either with its desire to preserve some degree of the status quo or with its predilection for the indirect approach to major change — making smaller changes to attain large ones.

The Role of Leadership

Leadership is the quality that is capable of motivating the membership to serve. The basic desire to perform a service, which attracted members to the auxiliary in the first place, is transformed into a program of action under leadership's skilled tutelage. In accepting this role, those in leadership positions assume certain responsibilities.

The first is to develop and maintain an atmosphere that is conducive to the personal growth of members as contributing individuals and that encourages optimal use of the human resources they represent. How well the auxiliary leader succeeds depends upon her ability to establish operational goals, fashion a sensible and responsive organization, and create a climate of trust and confidence.

Establishing Operational Goals

The auxiliary's ultimate goal, or purpose, provides an overall sense of direction. It is, however, nonoperational, for people find it difficult to measure progress toward an abstract concept that is constantly beyond reach. A nonoperational goal produces only frustration and disturbance in the group that is asked to achieve it.

The wise leader accepts the auxiliary's broad statement of purpose as an indicator of general direction and then establishes subgoals that, though clearly consistent with the ultimate purpose, *are* operational.

An example may be helpful. The auxiliary's purpose is stated as: "To render service to (name of health care institution) and its patients, and to assist (name of health care institution) in promoting the health and welfare of the community in accordance with objectives established by the institution" (Appendix A). This is the ultimate but nonoperational goal. More practical in terms of an operational goal would be encouraging the membership to create and implement a health education program for patients through the use of closed-circuit television. The members can visualize how they must proceed to meet this goal and also can evaluate the success of their efforts by the reaction of patients and staff.

Committees or task forces within the auxiliary can become disturbed, frustrated, and therefore nonproductive, unless their group goals have clearly defined limits. For instance, a puppet-making group is asked to create enough puppets for every first-time pediatrics patient entering the hospital in the coming year. But how many is "enough"?

Fashioning a Sensible and Responsive Organization

An auxiliary leader is obligated to live with and within the existing formal organization, but she is equally obligated to encourage or promote change in this organization, if change will produce a structure that makes more sense.

In creating an organization that meets the criteria for sensibility in basic structure and operations and responsiveness to the changing needs of its institution and community, an individual in a leadership position should attempt to fashion an auxiliary that is governed by bylaws uniquely its own, consistent with its purpose and responsibilities, and subject to frequent review; one in which lines of responsibility and authority, within the auxiliary and between the auxiliary and its institution, are clearly drawn and consistently observed; one that achieves a balance between democratic decision making and efficiency of operation; and one that is cognizant of its obligations to its members, committed to a program of leadership development, and able to adapt to changing situations through innovation and flexibility.

Creating a Climate of Trust and Confidence

A productive climate, in which members of the auxiliary work together creatively in an atmosphere of mutual trust and confidence, requires that certain conditions prevail. The organization must be capable of satisfying some basic needs of the individual members — most important, a sense of security, which comes from belonging to and acceptance by the group, and a need for appreciation.

In addition, the individual should feel free to express ideas without fear of reprisal if they differ from those of the power structure and should be able to make mistakes without fear of censure. In a productive climate, a premium is placed on the worth of ideas, rather than on the status of the person who expresses them.

A productive climate is not, it should be understood, necessarily synonymous with constant accord. Honest differences of opinion can contribute to growth, and there should be room in every auxiliary for a loyal opposition that makes its views known and then abides gracefully by majority decision.

A final condition is that when leadership delegates authority to get a job done, it also implicitly expresses trust that the job will be done.

Whether these conditions successfully prevail depends upon leadership's ability to make them a reality through appropriate attitudes, actions, and words. Indeed, a leader's attitudes and actions often are far more meaningful than her words. The effective leader is one who has learned how to nurture the conditions that instill trust and confidence in the membership and, simultaneously, how to use conflict creatively.

Other responsibilities of the auxiliary leadership include planning, coordinating, and evaluating the total program of assistance to the institution; and representing the auxiliary to its institution and to the community. Because of its influence on the organization's internal climate and program of action, leadership shapes the image of the auxiliary in the eyes of institution and community alike — a significant responsibility that leaders must constantly keep in mind.

Leadership Skills

Just as patterns of behavior can be developed or changed, so certain skills that are important in working with people can be learned.

Foremost among the skills required of leadership is the ability to communicate — to send and receive messages. The effective leader is aware that words, spoken or written, are not the sole means of communicating; messages are also sent or received, often unconsciously, by means of vocal inflections, gestures, facial expressions, and body movements. She soon learns that the test of effective communication lies not only in sending and receiving, but also in understanding the messages exchanged. She learns, too, that the ability to listen empathetically is by far the most valuable skill she can acquire.

Another skill is the art of timing, in presenting ideas for projects or new concepts of operation to membership. Appropriate timing can often mean the difference between a project's success or failure, between acceptance or rejection of a proposed change.

Additional skills that are particularly useful to the auxiliary leader include the ability to: delegate authority and then refrain from interfering in its exercise; anticipate the probable results of actions before making decisions; and be realistic about the capabilities of the organization and its members, as well as the limitations or possibilities inherent in every action taken.

It should be remembered, too, that friendliness is one of the greatest attributes an auxiliary leader can have.

Positions of Leadership

The evolution of leadership from membership is the result of a growth process. It is sustained by an auxiliary dedicated to fulfilling the requirements of leadership development.

The first requirement has to do with assigning members to committees or services. Through such assignments, individuals begin to acquaint themselves with the work of the auxiliary and, at the same time, have an opportunity to demonstrate their skills and capabilities. Assignments should be made with a knowledge of individual aptitudes and job requirements, imagination, and willingness to try and sometimes to err.

A new member who seems ideally suited to work on a particular committee can fail to meet expectations. In such a case, reassignment is always worth while. Similarly, despite the best intentions in the world, mistakes can be made in assigning new or additional responsibilities to members who have seemingly proved themselves, only to have them perform disappointingly.

In each case, the possible reasons for failure should be considered before any final estimate of a given member's leadership potential is made. Perhaps the member was uncomfortable in the group to which she was assigned, or the job failed to provide sufficient challenge. Perhaps she was not ready for a new post and needed more experience, or her interests were specialized and did not conform to her assignment, or she had no real desire for greater responsibility.

The second requirement is that the member should generally be given responsibility on a graduated basis. She should be asked to assume larger tasks when she has proved herself in smaller ones. On the other hand, an auxilian who has demonstrated her capacity to move to a larger arena of effort should not be kept waiting; her enthusiasm and interest may wane.

A third requirement has to do with training positions. (Training positions for officers' posts are discussed in the following section, "The Leadership Group.") *It is also essential that there be a training position, which carries the title of vice chairman, for every standing committee chairman.* This vice chairmanship is the final and vitally important rung prior to entry into the auxiliary's leadership group. Each vice chairman should be expected to assume responsibility for a segment of the committee's action program and should be consulted frequently by the chairman. In this way, the vice chairman can gain the experience she needs to move into the chairmanship, can demonstrate her abilities, and can help to relieve the chairman's load of responsibility. In turn, the auxiliary is given a real opportunity to evaluate each vice chairman's skills.

Although small auxiliaries may experience some problems in adopting this method of leadership training, some degree of adherence should be achieved as a means of ensuring high-quality leadership on a continuing basis.

Another requirement concerns participation in educational activities. Intra-auxiliary workshops and training sessions, as well as educational programs sponsored by other agencies, have an important place in leadership development. The coffee shop committee that sponsors regular discussion sessions for the shop's volunteers is assisting in the process of leadership development: Similarly, the committee chairman who seems to have presidential potential, or a newly elected vice president, should be given the opportunity to attend state or national hospital association institutes and conferences as well as local educational meetings. Through participation, they can gain much that will help them grow as individuals and, simultaneously, that will benefit the auxiliary. It is an unimaginative and limited policy that restricts such opportunities to the auxiliary's top officials.

A realistic approach to the amount of responsibility that leadership is expected to assume is also an important requirement. When the work of the auxiliary is so distributed that a disproportionate share falls on any one group or leader, an obstacle to leadership development is immediately created. Many potential leaders have become auxiliary dropouts because their responsibilities assumed overwhelming proportions. Therefore, in order to arrive at an equitable balance, the auxiliary that is dedicated to encouraging the growth of new leadership should carefully examine its operating structure and those provisions of the bylaws relating to officers and their responsibilities.

Finally, evaluation should be built into the auxiliary's leadership development program, in order to strengthen it and make it a pervasive influence that is felt throughout the organization. (See Chapter 11, "Planning and Evaluation.")

The Leadership Group
Board of Directors

The auxiliary's board of directors has the overall and ultimate responsibility for directing the affairs of the organization on behalf of the total membership and in the interests of the institution. One of its major tasks is to identify the primary objectives and essential functions of the auxiliary and to create related committees to perform certain of these functions. Accordingly, the board expresses its authority in a dual way: by accepting from the membership those responsibilities innate to any governing body, and by assigning responsibility to others for implementing action programs and certain functions related to the self-maintenance of the auxiliary. (See Chapter 5, "Committees.")

In fulfilling its obligations as a governing body, the board oversees long-range and current planning, so that the auxiliary's total program continues to progress in harmony with its overall purpose; sets objectives that accord with these plans and coordinates the activities of those to whom it assigns committee responsibilities; constantly reviews and evaluates the auxiliary's performance as well as its progress; and formulates policies to guide the membership in carrying out its programs.

Policy formulation, which is always conducted at the board level, provides officers and committee chairmen with an official frame of reference for decision making and efficient management. All such policy matters should be clearly and briefly stated in the administrative policies and procedures (see Chapter 4, "Organizational Principles"), to ensure uniform interpretation of policy and standardization of action at all levels within the auxiliary. The board should, of course, remain flexible regarding policy. Whenever a particular rule or regulation proves to be outdated, irrelevant, or cumbersome, it should be promptly reexamined from the viewpoint of change.

If the board is to fulfill its responsibilities, it must be structured as a "working board," including among its members only officers and standing committee chairmen. Of course, this concept must be established in the bylaws.

Upon occasion, department heads from the institution may be invited to attend board meetings when matters relating to their specific departments are under discussion, or when the board wishes to seek their advice on proposals. Such invitations go far toward strengthening communication and cementing relationships between the staff of the institution and the auxiliary. However, the auxiliary should under no circumstances dilute the board's strength, or seek to remedy a shaky relationship, by granting board membership of any kind to a department head.

Ad hoc committee chairmen are not members of the board of directors. Although they hold temporarily important posts, their positions cannot be described as essential, in the true sense of the word, nor do they have responsibility for an ongoing program. They should, however, be invited to sit in on board meetings when their committees' tasks are under discussion and should personally present their committees' final reports and recommendations to the board.

President

The president holds the top leadership post. This position of great authority is usually held by someone who has demonstrated her ability to wield a commensurate influence. She sets the tone of the auxiliary and, to a great extent, its current course of action. Maintaining a close working relationship with the institution's chief executive is, of course, among her primary responsibilities.

President-Elect

The person who occupies this position is officially designated as the successor at the end of the current president's term. This provision ensures continuity of leadership from one president to the next. However, to also ensure such continuity *during* the president's term, the president-elect should, in addition, be designated as the person to assume the presidency *at any time,* should the current president be absent or unable to continue in office.

Because the progressive auxiliary must satisfy — in ways that leave little to chance — the demands for leadership training as well as continuity in leadership, the president-elect should be given specific responsibilities. The person occupying this position should be considered the president's senior assistant and charged with coordinating those committees that are concerned with the self-maintenance functions of the auxiliary, such as membership relations, membership education, and financial planning. (See Chapter 5, "Committees," for a description of self-maintenance functions.) Such responsibilities will give the president-elect an opportunity to gain valuable experience in managing the affairs of the auxiliary and insight into those functions that are fundamental to the auxiliary's effectiveness.

Vice Presidents

Vice presidents are the president's lieutenants and potential successors. The need to spread the executive work load and the importance of developing new leadership on a continuous basis are both excellent reasons for having at least two vice presidents in addition to the president-elect: a vice president for community relations and a vice president for service. These officers assist the president, freeing her to concentrate on representing the auxiliary to the institution and the community.

It should be emphasized that this division of all activities within the auxiliary into the two categories of community relations and service is meant as a broad delineation, which probably should be sufficient to encompass the functions of today's auxiliary. However, as the auxiliary and its institution expand their visions of the auxiliary's role and major new areas of responsibility are assumed, additional vice presidents can be appointed to coordinate these functions. One such area might be the auxiliary's legislative action program.

The auxiliary that seeks the best in leadership must remain flexible in the matter of vice presidential succession, realizing that mistakes can be made and that situations change. In selecting its vice presidents, the organization should commit itself only to offering opportunities for further leadership development. By giving functional assignments and titles to its vice presidents, the auxiliary ensures that each vice president will, in fact, have a chance to demonstrate her leadership ability and gain broad experience. At the same time, the auxiliary avoids the danger always inherent in the numbering system, which often produces the assumption that each vice president moves up automatically until she reaches the presidency.

Secretaries, Treasurers, and Assistants

Because the positions of secretary and treasurer are somewhat specialized, the auxiliary may overlook the potential of these persons for eventually assuming other leadership positions. There is no logical reason that a competent secretary or treasurer cannot become an equally competent president — if given the opportunity for broader experience and additional training.

Whether or not these officers move up in position, they are bound to move out, in time, if the auxiliary adheres to the necessary revitalizing policy of limited tenure of office. The requirement that there be assistant officers in training ensures the important replacement personnel and, simultaneously, adds another dimension to the auxiliary's method of leadership development. The training program should include assignment of a specific portion of the work to the assistant, so that she will feel she is participating while she is learning.

Committee Chairmen

Committee chairmen are the action people within the auxiliary. They also represent its immediate reservoir of future top leadership. The importance of this group to the leadership team is discussed in Chapter 5, "Committees."

Authority and Influence

Not all persons in positions of authority in the auxiliary exercise influence and, conversely, not all persons who exercise influence hold positions of authority. Most auxiliaries have had at least one president who exercised no influence at all, and the leadership in many auxiliaries has had the experience of at least once coping with a member who held no position of authority but exercised great influence.

Similarly, mention should be made of the informal communications network that exists in every organization. The organizational structure establishes a formal channel of communication, but there is always an informal route. Leadership should learn to take advantage of this fact of organizational life and make constructive use of informal communication to weld the membership more closely together. On the other hand, leadership should remain aware that it is often through out-of-channels communication that influence without authority makes itself felt.

Use of Past Leadership

The auxiliary that is concerned with developing future leadership is equally concerned with the wise use of past leadership. Past presidents, in particular, possess valuable knowledge and experience that should be fully utilized. However, the auxiliary should avoid placing a past president in any position that would conflict with the current president's authority or freedom to function. Even with the best intentions, an immediate past president may feel the need to "keep her hand in" the management of the current president's responsibilities.

It is advisable, therefore, not to include the immediate past president on the board of directors during the year following her term of office. This arrangement permits the new president to more completely express her personal interpretation of the president's role and to develop independence in making decisions. To be an effective leader, she needs room to expand, to experiment, to make mistakes, and to achieve success on the basis of her own ability. Should she desire the help and advice of her predecessor, as well she may, she should consider this as a voluntary decision rather than an obligation.

Several highly suitable positions within the auxiliary make productive use of a past president's expertise, without requiring board membership. Serving as chairman of the nominating committee, a key post, is one possibility. Another is chairmanship of or membership on an ad hoc committee. An ad hoc committee is appointed for a particular short-term task, usually one of immediate importance. A past president would seem especially appropriate as the auxiliary's representative to another community organization, a post of prestige and importance. Or, she may prefer the relative quiet of membership on the committee of her choice. Whatever the solution, it should enable the immediate past president to remain active, interested, and useful without infringing on the prerogatives of the current president.

In the final analysis, the decision as to the best use of the immediate past president resides with the individual auxiliary. It is recommended that the immediate past president be encouraged to serve in a position not carrying board membership. This recommendation is based on the valid arguments advanced above. If an auxiliary should take the opposing view, it should be aware of the reasons behind its decision and be able to support it with equally strong arguments.

Others who have held leadership positions within the auxiliary, such as vice presidents or committee chairmen, also have much to contribute to the auxiliary's future. Their talents and experience should not be overlooked nor their usefulness and enthusiasm allowed to dissipate because of lack of involvement in auxiliary affairs.

chapter 4
Organizational Principles

Good bylaws are the foundation upon which sound
auxiliary organization rests. Bylaws provide a portrait of the
group, for merely by reading them, one can discern the
nature and character of the auxiliary organization.

Mrs. Harry Milton,
former chairman,
Council on Hospital Auxiliaries
(now Committee on Volunteers),
American Hospital Association

Formal organization is the means by which the auxiliary, as a
responsible entity, establishes its relationship to its institution
and its legal personality, ensures its continuity, and formalizes
its purpose. Thus, planning for auxiliary organization involves
consideration of its legal status and of basic principles of organization.

Legal Personality

An auxiliary is a legal entity from the inception of
its formal organization. It falls on those responsible for its formal organization to choose the most appropriate legal form for
its existence.

Because the entire subject of legal considerations is handled
in Chapter 6, it suffices to say here that it is preferable for an
auxiliary to be legally organized as an integral part of its parent
institution. This legal relationship to the institution should be

indicated clearly in the auxiliary's bylaws and confirmed by formal action of the institution's governing authority.

Purpose

Because organizational structure (bylaws and administrative policies and procedures) is the medium by which an auxiliary accomplishes its purpose, the more accurately this structure reflects the purpose of the auxiliary, the higher the level of accomplishment in realizing goals.

The auxiliary's statement of purpose should serve as a means of measuring the adequacy of its organization. This statement proclaims the reason for the auxiliary's existence and acknowledges the ultimate authority of the institution.

Authority and Accountability

The individuals or the group empowered to exercise authority on behalf of an organization should be identified and the scope of that authority delineated in the formal instrument of organization — the bylaws.

The auxiliary's authority is essentially a delegated authority. In authorizing the establishment of an auxiliary, the institution's governing body in effect delegates to the auxiliary certain powers. (See Chapter 2, "The Auxiliary's Accountabilities and Relationships.") At the same time, the governing body retains the right to review and approve activities and programs conducted by the auxiliary for the institution. Both the delegation of authority and the restrictions on its use should be reflected in the auxiliary's bylaws.

When the institution delegates authority to an auxiliary, it is vesting power, in a general sense, in the membership. However, this authority is actually exercised by the auxiliary's board of directors, which is empowered to do so by the membership, through the auxiliary's bylaws.

Inherent in any delegation of authority is the requirement of accountability for the use of that authority. Thus, the auxiliary's board is accountable to the membership and to the institution for the exercise of the authority expressly delegated to it. And the auxiliary, as a whole, must hold itself accountable to the institution and, specifically, to the institution's chief executive, for such authority as remains vested in the membership.

Communications

The organizational structure should provide for a formal communications network. Principles of organization dictate that communications at the highest level between auxiliary and institution should be channeled between the auxiliary president and the chief executive and his staff. Furthermore, any communications between the auxiliary and the department heads of the institution should flow through the administration, unless the administration authorizes a more direct route. Communications within the auxiliary also should travel through channels established by the organizational structure.

Bylaws

Bylaws are the auxiliary's expression of formal organization; they also represent agreement among the members as to regulation of the auxiliary's internal affairs and its relationships to others. The bylaws establish the basic policies under which the auxiliary must operate unless, and until, membership agrees to change them.

Because the bylaws mirror the character of the auxiliary and establish its organizational framework and its organic structure, any decisions that are incorporated into articles of the bylaws must be made in full recognition of the purpose and responsibilities of the auxiliary. These decisions always should be made in consultation with the institution's administration.

As a legal instrument, bylaws are made to be observed. They are also a dynamic instrument that must change and grow if they are to reflect the growth of the auxiliary as it adapts to meet the evolving needs of its institution and the community. Conversely, bylaws that are in a perpetual state of change and amendment are probably too restrictive and cluttered with details and therefore interfere with efficient operation.

Administrative Policies and Procedures

Supplementing the bylaws are the administrative policies and procedures, which represent an expansion and replacement of what are sometimes known as "standing rules." The administrative policies and procedures incorporate decisions made by the auxiliary's board on methods for the administration of the basic policies in the bylaws, and they may not supersede the authority established in the bylaws.

They are, however, more flexible than the bylaws, because they can be changed by action of the auxiliary's board, without referral to the total membership or to the institution's administration. They also have the advantage of making it unnecessary to provide in the bylaws for most procedural details, particularly those likely to require rather frequent alteration. This eliminates the obvious hazard of continually having to change the bylaws as new situations arise.

Model Bylaws

The model bylaws in Appendix A are based upon the concepts and recommendations expressed in this book. It is hoped that they will be helpful to established auxiliaries in meeting the challenge of change, as well as to auxiliaries in the formative stage. The following bylaws sections are of particular importance.

Statement of Purpose

This statement, discussed briefly at the beginning of this chapter, should reflect recognition of the major changes occurring in health care institutions. Such changes, which affect all parts of the institution, including the auxiliary, are a response to technological advances and increasing emphasis on the responsibility of health care institutions in meeting the needs of their communities. Consequently, the American Hospital Association recommends that the traditional definition of auxiliary purpose, usually stated as "To render service to_____Hospital and its patients," be expanded to read: "To render service to (name of health care institution) and its patients and to assist (name of health care institution) in promoting the health and welfare of the community in accordance with objectives established by the institution" (Appendix A).

Open Membership

By providing that membership is open to all adults interested in the institution and willing to uphold the auxiliary's purpose, the bylaws (1) acknowledge the right of the community to participate in an organization that it is asked to support,

(2) indicate an awareness that the auxiliary is a component part of a community institution, and (3) provide the health care institution with a link to *all* segments of the community it serves.

Fiscal Policies

The bylaws provisions regarding fiscal policies should (1) distinguish between auxiliary funds and earnings, (2) provide for a budget, (3) require annual audited financial reports, and (4) require that all auxiliary contracts with outside agencies be countersigned by the appropriate institution official and that all auxiliary bank accounts be established by resolution of the institution's governing authority.

Executive Power

The bylaws provision establishing the powers of the board of directors should state clearly and unequivocally that the board shall administer the affairs of the auxiliary on behalf of the membership and in a manner consistent with the bylaws. It should state with equal clarity that board actions, other than those concerning the auxiliary's internal affairs, are subject to the approval of the institution's governing body or its representative, the chief executive.

Structural Committees

Only the nominating committee and the executive committee (if one exists) should be described in the bylaws. These are structural committees. Standing committees should be described in the administrative policies and procedures, so that bylaws revisions will not be required as committee duties develop and change from year to year.

Executive Committee

The executive committee, formed within the auxiliary's board of directors, is empowered, within certain limitations, to act for the board. If it is to exist at all, it can exist only as part of the auxiliary's legal structure, and therefore must be designated and described in the bylaws.

Although an executive committee may be superfluous when the board of directors is small, it performs a very useful function when the auxiliary is governed by a large board. The committee not only can serve as an advisory group to the president, but also can be assembled easily in case emergency action is necessary. However, the board of directors should take serious exception to too frequent "emergency" meetings of the executive committee, for they may indicate that the board, the legitimate executive arm of the organization, is being bypassed and its rightful power usurped.

Nominating Committee

Whatever the size of the auxiliary, parliamentary procedure demands a nominating committee, which must be named and described in the bylaws.

No one has yet devised the perfect composition for a nominating committee. The model bylaws in Appendix A make yet another attempt and succeed in incorporating a number of valid principles, all of which are described in the comment following Article X, Section 3.

Regardless of the committee's composition, many auxiliaries encounter difficulty in persuading their nominating committees to seriously assume responsibility for year-round effort. This is a grave problem indeed, for it can hamper the auxiliary's leadership development program.

Two things can help overcome this difficulty. The first is a bylaws section that provides for (1) automatic appointment of the immediate past president as committee chairman and (2) election, on a rotating basis, of four of the five other members. Thus, five-sixths of the committee's complement is named at the start of the auxiliary's year. The second is the simple device of preparing a written description of precisely what is expected of the committee.

Normal expectations for a nominating committee should include: that the committee meet at regular intervals to consider possible candidates for elective positions; that it meet periodically with the membership relations committee to gather suggestions; that the chairman report from time to time, and at the request of the president, to the auxiliary's board; that the committee be aware of and take into consideration a possible conflict of interest before making a nomination; and that the committee maintain appropriate records.

In order to avoid a possible conflict of interest, the nominating committee should consider a nominee in light of all her roles in life — not only her role as an auxilian but also as someone with home or career responsibilities and perhaps other volunteer commitments.

It should be noted that membership on this committee does not preclude an individual's eligibility for nomination to an office within the auxiliary.

The records kept by the committee should contain the type of information that will be of continuing assistance to the committee as time passes and that will also help the auxiliary president seeking potential candidates for appointive posts.

This written statement of expectations should be in the hands of all members of the nominating committee, and as a matter of routine copies should be given to new chairmen as they take over and to new nominees when they are asked to serve.

Subgroups—An Organizational Vehicle

When a health care institution serves an area composed of several communities, or a widespread geographical area, it may be necessary and desirable to establish subgroups of the auxiliary, sometimes known as "twig" groups, one for each community or section. Such subgroups frequently can resolve the organizational problems that stem from spreading the auxiliary's manpower too thinly over too much territory or in too many programs. The result of effectively using subgroups can be better provision of service to more people. Another advantage of establishing subgroups is the opportunity to conduct expanded membership drives, thus getting more of the community actively involved in serving the institution through an increase in membership. With additional membership, the auxiliary's diversity of talent should also increase.

The following information concerning the structure and functions of subgroups represents a suggested approach for auxiliaries wishing to establish such entities or to reorganize those already in existence.

Membership in a subgroup would naturally include membership in the parent body of the auxiliary. There is no separate auxiliary membership in addition to subgroup membership. Thus, an individual participates in the work of the auxiliary as a member of a subgroup.

All subgroups of an auxiliary are governed by the auxiliary's bylaws. Each subgroup has its own president and such other officers as size and program dictate. They are elected annually, with the president of the subgroup serving as a member of the auxiliary's board of directors. Where necessary, subgroups may be authorized to appoint committees.

Subgroups support the auxiliary's programs and projects, but also function independently, conducting their own activities that have been approved by the auxiliary's board. They can also work with other subgroups on projects. Coordination of programs between subgroups, and between subgroups and the parent auxiliary, is the responsibility of the auxiliary's board of directors. Each subgroup holds its own meetings when desired. In addition, there should be several general membership meetings of the auxiliary scheduled yearly, open to members of all subgroups.

Regarding the handling of money, all membership dues and earnings of subgroups should be paid into the main treasury of the auxiliary. Each subgroup will then be given necessary operating funds on the basis of an annual budget approved by the auxiliary's board of directors.

Subgroups represent an organizational alternative to the auxiliary that is experiencing difficulty in operating under the traditional single group form. In the interests of serving its institution and community at large to the best of its ability, such an auxiliary should be willing to explore the possibilities of the subgroup concept.

Adaptation to Change

As new organizational forms for health care delivery and new methods of financing health care evolve, hospitals are modifying their own organizational structures to meet these changes. The auxiliary, in turn, experiences — directly or indirectly — the effects of any changes undergone by its institution and must modify its own organizational structure and programs accordingly.

The pressures being applied today by federal, state, and local governments and by the community to cut the costs of health care while continuing to improve its delivery have motivated hospitals to seek alternative organizational arrangements to meet this challenge. As hospitals explore new approaches to providing health services, they look to mergers and other forms of hospital systems as possible ways of maximizing resources, coordinating services, containing costs, and improving the quality of patient care.

Mergers and Consolidations

When it becomes apparent to two or more health care institutions, usually within the same community, that they can better provide health care services by combining their efforts and resources, a merger may be effected. Under this arrangement, the institutions join together under a single corporate entity and name — usually the name of one of the institutions. A merger generally occurs when one institution assumes the assets and liabilities of another. The merger may be a corporate one only, with each institution maintaining its own, original physical unit, or it may be an actual physical merger as well as a corporate one, with both institutions joined within the existing physical plant of one of them or both moving into an entirely different facility. Mergers can occur between similar institutions, such as two or more short-term acute care hospitals, or between institutions that have different purposes, such as a short-term acute care hospital combining with a specialty hospital, a rehabilitation center, an extended care facility, or a freestanding neighborhood clinic.

Consolidation is another organizational device being utilized by institutions. Consolidation consists of two or more institutions dissolving their corporate identities and establishing a new and separate corporation that assumes all the assets and liabilities of the original institutions.

The implications for the auxiliaries attached to institutions that have merged or consolidated can be considerable in terms of organizational structure, purpose, and program. A situation of multiple auxiliaries can result, with multiple identities, goals, interests, and methods of operating. In order to avoid working at cross purposes, duplicating efforts, and becoming rivals that compete for recognition from the institution and the community, these auxiliaries should merge to support a common cause when their institutions merge or consolidate.

Auxiliaries should regard organizational changes of their institutions as prime opportunities to increase the scope and effectiveness of their service. By joining forces, auxiliaries can multiply their manpower, money, time, and talent, utilizing these resources to the greatest advantage of the institutions involved.

Mrs. Newton Millham, former chairman of the American Hospital Association Committee on Volunteers, in discussing the auxiliary's attitude toward a merger of its institution and the question of where the auxiliary's loyalty lies, states: "When, after careful consideration, it has been decided that the hospital can better carry out its purpose of providing the best care possible for its community through a merger, the auxiliary is committed to accept its new role and to work for the best interests of the new entity" (ref. 34). The term "committed" is the operative word regarding the appropriate attitude for the auxiliary.

When a merger or consolidation is being negotiated, it is helpful to the auxiliaries involved if the presidents of each group are kept informed about the proceedings from the very beginning. This is important if the line of communication between institution and auxiliary is to be used most effectively. Without inclusion in the information process, the auxiliaries may believe that they are unimportant in the total institutional picture. Further, such information helps to orient auxiliary leadership to the various steps involved in the specific merger or consolidation, preparing them to better educate their membership and the community about the coming event. In the area of community education, it can be especially important to provide advance information about a potential merger, particularly if it involves a change in location for the institution, or major alterations in types of services. Such new arrangements can be disturbing to a community that has come to depend upon certain established patterns of health care delivery. Although in many instances the institution automatically includes the auxiliary in this educational process, there may be times when the auxiliary will have to take the initiative itself and request that its representatives be kept informed as to the merger proceedings.

As the merger becomes imminent, the time is also propitious for the affected auxiliaries to sit down together and determine their joint future on behalf of their institutions. It is a time for a comprehensive evaluation of each auxiliary's goals and operations and for the development of an imaginative plan to channel these diverse interests into a coordinated, effective, and workable force for their institutions. Legal reorganization will, of course, be mandatory as well, if multiple auxiliaries are to become one. In essence, a new auxiliary is being created, but with the advantage of past experience to guide it. Such initiatives will be taken, of course, with the full knowledge of the institutions involved.

To smooth the transition, it may be wise to enlist the assistance of an outside consultant who can provide organizational and managerial expertise. As a matter of course, the institutions' attorneys should also be consulted as to legal ramifications, such as determination of the legal status of the new auxiliary in relation to the institution, development of new bylaws, and related matters.

The actual merging or consolidation of the auxiliaries should be conducted on a well-planned, step-by-step basis. The process could be initiated by holding meetings of each auxiliary's membership group in order to communicate information about the merger proceedings, to obtain support for the combining of the auxiliaries, and to gain membership's approval for each auxiliary's board of directors to appoint representatives to a combined steering or coordinating committee.

The steering committee should include representatives of the leadership and the general membership from each auxiliary. The initial meeting of the steering committee should be an orientation session during which representatives of the administrations of the merging institutions offer insights into the reasons for the merger and discuss the role of the auxiliary that will be serving this new entity.

Subsequent meetings of the steering committee should be devoted to the following activities:

- Identifying the needs of the new institution in terms of programs, services, and funds.
- Defining the institution's expectations of the new auxiliary — particularly those expectations that may not have been fulfilled by the separate auxiliaries.
- Reviewing the background of each auxiliary, its current programs and projects.
- Discussing similarities and differences among the groups.

- Discussing how to utilize each auxiliary's present leadership in such a way that there is no loss of prestige.
- Defining to the auxiliaries the advantages of merging.
- Establishing the overall purpose and specific objectives of the new auxiliary and possible new programs for the combined group. It could be helpful to emphasize that the objectives of the new organization can encompass those of the previous auxiliaries — when appropriate — and perhaps revitalize the membership, presenting new opportunities for meaningful service and projects.
- Creating an organizational structure and bylaws for the new auxiliary. The steering committee should appoint a bylaws committee for this purpose, composed of several representatives from each auxiliary. The institutions' attorneys should be invited to act as consultants to the committee. It is suggested that the bylaws committee utilize the model bylaws in Appendix A of this manual, as well as information on organizational principles, in developing recommendations to present to the steering committee.
- Planning for the election of new officers for the combined auxiliary. A nominating committee, composed of individuals from each of the participating auxiliaries, should be appointed by the steering committee to fulfill this charge.

It is also important that representatives of the steering committee meet periodically with their respective administrations to report on progress and that they keep their individual auxiliaries regularly informed of plans for the merger.

Procedures for accomplishing the actual merger of the auxiliaries should be worked out with legal advice. Provision will have to be made for the membership to approve the bylaws and slate of officers and to take whatever legal action is needed to dissolve the existing groups and form the new group. Members become charter members of the new auxiliary, and this charter membership can be kept open for several months to encourage others in the community to join. The establishment of the new organization offers an excellent opportunity for membership recruitment, which should be fully utilized by the combined auxiliary.

If the administration is strongly committed to the need for a unified auxiliary, and will support the efforts of the individual groups to unite, the transition period leading to the merger of the auxiliaries will be more easily facilitated. This *can* be a sensitive time for the groups involved, particularly those with strong identities. Fear of being submerged and losing the identity that has taken so long to establish can be a very real concern for the auxiliaries. The leadership of the auxiliaries should emphasize that it will attempt to retain the best characteristics of each group, incorporating these positive features into the structure and program of the new entity.

Shared Services

A contemporary method of health care delivery, shared services can be described as "the wide range of different ways in which health care institutions can cooperate to care for patients. Medical specialists, equipment and facilities, personnel, and the performance of services are all elements which may be involved in a sharing arrangement. In fact, almost any hospital activity can be carried out on a shared basis. . . . Although hospitals come first to mind when shared services are considered, opportunities exist for other health care institutions as well. Extended care facilities, nursing homes, clinics and other institutions can often share services, either among themselves or with nearby hospitals" (ref. 61).

In essence, then, shared services are those clinical or administrative facilities that are common to two or more organizations and that are used jointly or cooperatively by them in some way for the purpose of improving services and containing cost.

Some examples of services that can be shared by health care institutions are obstetrical, radiological, emergency, laboratory, and laundry services, which eliminate the need for neighboring hospitals to maintain similar departments that duplicate functions. Other sharing possibilities include computerized information services (data processing), insurance programs, management consulting services, and inservice education and training programs.

Auxiliaries serving health care institutions that have these types of sharing arrangements may want to reassess their programs of volunteer service and financial assistance in view of these interrelationships. If a hospital and a nursing home share some kinds of services on a daily basis, for example, the auxiliary might consider a program of service to the nursing home in addition to its efforts for the hospital. This could include regular visitation to residents by auxilians, assistance in conducting recreational therapy and reality orientation programs, provision of entertainment expenses and transportation for residents' outside activities, and financial aid for the purpose of establishing specific programs for residents. The morale boosting generated by such auxiliary activities can be immeasurable for these individuals who often feel forgotten. In addition, community relations can be enhanced by the auxiliary's interest and effort on behalf of another community institution.

chapter 5
Committees

'A committee is a group of the unfit trying to lead
the unwilling to do the unnecessary.' But joke if you must,
the committee is here to stay. Despite its weaknesses
at the hands of leaders and members, we can't
carry on our political, social, religious,
and economic business without it.

For Those Who Must Lead . . .
The Hillsdale College Leadership Letter,
"The Care and Feeding of Committees,"
2:1, Dec. 1963.

Why is it that some auxiliaries always seem to accomplish what
they set out to do with relative speed and ease, whereas others
are notable only for their good intentions? The answer lies in
the presence — or absence — of a rational, flexible system for
creating committees.

Committees are the action arm of the auxiliary — the media
through which programs are translated into reality. A rational
system for creating committees should have the capacity for
intelligent assignment of areas of responsibility and action. At
the same time, it should provide a mechanism for coordinating
all these activities, so that the auxiliary offers its institution a
unified and progressive program of service.

It is the responsibility of the auxiliary's board of directors,
guided by the bylaws, to establish a system for creating com-

mittees. (See Chapter 3 for a discussion on the authority of the auxiliary's board of directors.) The system chosen by the board is highly individualized, reflecting the auxiliary's own specific needs and those of the institution it serves. In addition, the system should be responsive, continually growing and changing to accommodate newly interpreted functions or new objectives of the auxiliary.

Self-Maintenance Functions

The board's first task is to identify the functions relating to the auxiliary's self-maintenance and to decide how responsibility for each shall be assigned.

Membership Relations

Members are crucial to both the auxiliary's existence and its capacity to serve; they represent its most valuable resource. Without question, activities relating to membership, and to individual members, comprise an essential function demanding special attention and warranting creation of a standing membership relations committee.

Recruitment is chief among the committee's responsibilities, but its effectiveness cannot be measured by numbers. Effective recruitment means more than simply adding people to the membership roster, willing though they may be to commit themselves to the purpose of the auxiliary. It means, more important in the long view, retaining recruited members and maintaining their active interest. Thus, this committee should assume much of the responsibility, on behalf of the auxiliary, for fulfilling the organization's obligations to its members, as discussed in Chapter 3, "Membership and Leadership."

In order to develop the kind of membership relations that produce dedicated volunteers, the committee demonstrates the auxiliary's concern for its individual members, thus playing a vital role in forging lifelong bonds between the organization and its membership. This concern is expressed through the use of certain techniques of relating to members, such as:

• Interviewing each new recruit and ascertaining her (his) needs and talents, thereby helping each to find meaningful participation in the affairs of the auxiliary.

- Continuing to keep an interest in each member, for the purpose of assisting the nominating committee, the president, and other committee chairmen in their search for specialized talents and potential leadership.

Education is the other principal activity relating to membership. It represents one of the auxiliary's major obligations to its members, and it is a primary motivating force in membership involvement.

Although there is a strong affinity between membership relations and membership education, the latter is so essential, both to the auxiliary's internal health and self-maintenance and to its external action program, that it merits appointment of a separate committee with its own representative on the board. The responsibilities of the membership education committee are discussed in detail in Chapter 8, "Education."

Leadership Development

Leadership has been described as a product of the auxiliary's concern for membership, and its development can be easily identified as a self-maintenance function. By its very nature, however, new leadership develops through the efforts of many facets of the auxiliary — the nominating committee, the officers, and various committee chairmen. All evaluate members' performances and assess leadership potential. In the final analysis, however, the board of directors assumes the ultimate responsibility for coordinating these diverse efforts and fostering the evolution of new leadership from the membership ranks.

Financial Planning

In view of its overall responsibility for managing the auxiliary's financial affairs, the board of directors has these broadly stated obligations: to account for the use of all funds entrusted to it; to use the income from dues wisely and for purposes consistent with the auxiliary's objectives; and to expend any funds raised from the general public for purposes that improve the institution's ability to render optimum care, on its own premises or within the community. The auxiliary's board of directors delegates the specific responsibility for implementing these functions to the finance committee.

The first obligation is met when the treasurer keeps accurate income and expenditure records and annually presents an audited financial report to the auxiliary's board. In order to fulfill its other obligations — ensuring the proper use of dues income and funds raised from the general public — the board must first distinguish between auxiliary funds and auxiliary earnings.

Auxiliary funds consist of membership dues, donor-restricted contributions,* and fees paid to attend auxiliary-sponsored educational meetings — all allocated for the purpose of running the auxiliary. Auxiliary earnings, on the other hand, consist of all monies derived from publicly supported auxiliary activities, including auxiliary-operated shops. The former represent an auxiliary resource and can be expended at the discretion of the board of directors for any purpose consistent with auxiliary objectives. The latter must be expended in ways that can be justified to the contributing public and that are authorized by the institution.

In summation, auxiliary funds and earnings differ in their sources, in the uses to which they may be properly channeled, and in the degree of control exercised by the board over their expenditure. Because auxiliary funds are necessary to the organization's self-maintenance and viability, they are obviously managed differently from auxiliary earnings, which are an aspect of the auxiliary's accountability (responsibility) to the community from which it is drawing these earnings.

In order to ensure that expenditures are consistent with the distinction between auxiliary funds and earnings, the board may want to discuss with the finance committee the feasibility of preparing two budgets: (1) an operating budget to maintain the auxiliary and (2) a financial contributions budget encompassing the fund-raising and related activities initiated by the auxiliary on behalf of its institution.

The finance committee develops the budgets on the basis of data gathered from the various committees. Each committee should be asked to estimate and justify its expenses for the coming year and to estimate any earnings it expects its activities to produce.

*Donor-restricted contributions are contributions that the donor restricts to the specified use by the auxiliary itself.

Operating Budget

In dollars and cents terms, the operating budget expresses the auxiliary's plan of operations for the coming year. As part of its budget-making responsibility, the finance committee should:

- Analyze costs, including the expense of "doing business," such as postage, printing, educational activities, awards, and auditing fees. Some auxiliaries may have unusual and additional expenses, such as the salary of an executive secretary. The cost of this salary should be included in developing a budget.

- Estimate income from dues, donor-restricted contributions, fees from meetings, and so forth.

- On the basis of these data, assist the board in establishing a final budget that is realistic, both financially and in terms of the year's program objectives. The final budget should also be sufficiently detailed to guide the treasurer in making disbursements (as provided in Appendix A, the model by-laws, Article VIII, Section 3, under "Comment").

A model operating budget is presented on page 56. The format of this budget, and of the financial contributions budget on page 58, is basically a categorical breakdown of the types of income and expenses most generally encountered by auxiliaries.

Traditionally, expenses connected with the attendance of auxilians at out-of-town educational meetings have been included, if at all, in the operating budget, as they are in the model. However, the operating budget, based primarily on income from dues that are often minimal, may be insufficient to support such expenses. If this is the case, the auxiliary may wish to consider an alternative method of financing the cost of special, continuing educational opportunities for auxilians.

Utilizing this method, the auxiliary, with the approval of the administration, would include monies to cover such educational expenses in its financial contributions budget as part of its contribution to the institution's program for continuing education. Expenditures for auxilians could be made only with the written approval of the appropriate person within the institution, who would have to review each request and agree upon the justification for the expense.

OPERATING BUDGET

Income

1. **Dues.**

2. Fees paid to attend auxiliary-sponsored educational seminars and related events.

3. Donor-restricted contributions, earmarked for designated use, from individuals and groups.

Expenses

1. Office: postage, printing, stationery, telephone, other supplies, secretarial and auditing expenses.

2. Educational meetings:
   a. Membership meetings: cost of film rentals, speakers' fees and expenses, refreshments, and so on.
   b. Special educational programs or meetings for auxilians: cost of film rentals, speakers' fees and expenses, and so forth.
   c. Out-of-town meetings: cost of transportation, lodging, food, registration fees at institutes and seminars, reimbursement for child care expenses, for persons who are attending such events in an official capacity and at the specific request of the auxiliary.

3. Awards for volunteer service: cost of pins or other tangible types of awards. This includes awards for auxilians and may include recognition of inservice volunteers.

4. Special functions: cost of giving a new members' reception or an orientation meeting prior to obtaining members' applications; special events parties for members, including affairs during annual meeting of auxiliary, holiday parties, and so on.

5. Contingency funds.

6. Publications of the auxiliary: cost of producing the members' newsletter and any other bulletins or related materials.

7. Dues for membership in state hospital associations and group membership in other community organizations.

8. Cost of subscriptions to relevant periodicals and newsletters, or the cost of purchasing books, for the use of membership.

When the institution assumes responsibility for such expenditures, it is stating, in effect, that it considers the auxiliary's service valuable to the institution, its patients, and the community. Consequently, it regards a continuing education program for auxilians as necessary as that for its employees.

Financial Contributions Budget

The auxiliary's plan for meeting its financial commitment to its institution during the coming year is reflected in a financial contributions budget. This projected budget also represents the board's attitude on fundamental questions of policy:

- In view of the auxiliary's purpose and objectives, what proportion of the membership's total effort, if any, should be expended in activities that produce funds for the institution?
- If the traditional fund-raising role is to be continued, what priorities have been established for the use of these funds? (See page 97.)

Other Financial Considerations

Retention of large amounts of money in the auxiliary's bank account can create tax problems, regardless of the reasons for accumulating funds. Some auxiliaries maintain contingency funds; others accumulate money for a specific purpose, such as a long-range project. Such practices can be dangerous for auxiliaries in relation to maintaining their tax-exempt status with the federal government. This is particularly relevant to separately incorporated auxiliaries or auxiliaries that are unincorporated associations.

Assume, for example, that a separately incorporated auxiliary is exempt from federal income tax under Section 501(c)(3) of the Internal Revenue Code. Unreasonable accumulation of funds could then be considered as not conforming to the original exempt purpose of the auxiliary, and the auxiliary's tax-exempt status could be revoked, subjecting the auxiliary to liability for back taxes. The auxiliary should consult its institution's attorney and accountant for the appropriate method of operation regarding this matter.

Action Programs

After successfully identifying the functions essential to the self-maintenance of the auxiliary, the board should

FINANCIAL CONTRIBUTIONS BUDGET
Net Income*

1. Fund-raising projects—Contributions.
   a. Thrift shops.
   b. Memorial funds.
   c. Special events of all kinds.
   d. Annual campaign for institution.
   e. Seed money for upcoming projects, derived from previous year's fund-raising efforts, and not expended at that time.
2. Fund-raising projects—Income-producing services.
   a. Gift and coffee shops.
   b. Television rental.
   c. Gift carts.
3. Interest on savings accounts.
   a. General funds.
   b. Contingency funds.

Distribution of Net Income

1. Contributions to institution.
   a. Regular gifts to maintain ongoing programs. Examples:
      (1) Continuing education for employees.
      (2) Financial aid to education for health careers for young people and others in the community.
      (3) Social service funds given to social service department of institution to help patients needing emergency money.
      (4) Subsidies for the department of volunteer services, to pay for uniforms, meals at institution, and transportation for inservice volunteers unable to meet expenses; money for inservice volunteer educational programs.
   b. Special gifts for ongoing programs and short-term projects; seed money for new programs.

---

*Net income is the figure arrived at after deducting expenses from the gross income obtained from fund-raising efforts.

Examples:
(1) Community education programs on general health issues, preventive health care, living with specific illnesses, and so on.
(2) Patients' library.

c. Expenditures for functions.

Examples:
(1) For employees and staff: conducting events for general employees and professional staff, such as holiday parties; receptions to welcome foreign doctors and their families, other new doctors, professional staff members, student nurses.
(2) For the institution: providing holiday decorations for public areas or patient areas; conducting open house and tour of the institution for the community, with refreshments.

2. Contributions to other community agencies (as approved by the institution).

Examples:
a. Contributions to such organizations as the Visiting Nurse Association, to provide funds for certain previously hospitalized patients who are being cared for at home.
b. Funds for halfway houses, to help former alcoholics, drug addicts, and individuals who have been hospitalized for mental problems, in readjusting to society.

look outward and determine the broad areas of need to be met if the auxiliary is to carry out its purpose: Can the institution benefit from a program of service to the hospital staff? Is there a role for the auxiliary in supporting national legislative programs? Should the auxiliary commit itself to more extensive participation in community health projects sponsored by other agencies?

Once these major areas of need have been pinpointed, the board should then ascertain the specific action programs — or responsibilities — the auxiliary will undertake within each area.

As an illustration, in discussing a program of service to the hospital staff, the board might review the problem of frequent absenteeism among female hospital employees. Investigation might indicate that a day care center for the children of these employees could help to resolve this situation. Through its committee structure, and with a well-defined plan, the auxiliary might work with the administration to locate space, staff, equipment, and necessary funds, thereby accepting specific responsibilities for a program of service to the hospital staff.

This recognition of an actual — and, in this case, immediate — need of its institution, and the action program necessary for its fulfillment, clearly illustrates how effectively an auxiliary can operate. However, projects should be realistically conceived, with the auxiliary responding to valid problems that are resolvable, to some degree, through its collective efforts.

In addition to determining the specific needs of its institution, the auxiliary's board should consider other important criteria before assigning responsibility for carrying out action programs. These criteria include the capabilities of the auxiliary membership, with emphasis on the specific talents of individuals; availability of leadership, personnel, and financial resources; availability of guidance and assistance from the institution's staff, when necessary; and the community's needs.

Prior to undertaking any major action programs for its institution, the auxiliary's board should submit such plans both to the institution's administration and appropriate staff and to the general membership of the auxiliary for final approval. In the latter instance, it is often difficult, and sometimes impossible, to obtain the necessary auxiliary support for projects without previously involving the potential "supporters" in the actual decision-making process.

Whatever differences may exist among auxiliaries regarding action committees, their structures and assignments, there is a meeting ground in the sharing of a common purpose and common functions. Accordingly, certain basic guidelines may prove helpful to the auxiliary as it develops committees to conduct its action programs.

1. *Create a standing committee only when it can be charged with the development and execution of a distinct action program and define its boundaries of responsibility with care and precision.*

As an example, the following profile of a community relations committee illustrates the effective and often complex ways in which a committee may serve its auxiliary.

The term *community relations* has received such wide and diverse use in recent years that it has become an all-encompassing phrase and, as such, is often confusing. As a concept specifically relating to auxiliaries, community relations means the auxiliary's participation in developing greater interaction between itself and the community and in performing the same function for its institution.

The first effort in opening up channels of communication with the community begins at home. However, the auxiliary needs to equate "community" with more than its own membership. Although this membership may be truly representative of its community (see Chapter 3, "Membership and Leadership," concerning composition of the auxiliary), a broader and more valid definition would include auxiliary members, nonmembers who come into contact with the institution and the auxiliary, and all other segments of society with whom contact is made. In this larger sense, a community relations committee becomes a necessity in implementing community interaction.

Logically, then, the community relations committee should be assigned broad responsibility for: (1) activities that reach out to the general public in presenting a picture of the institution; and (2) activities that use, in an appropriate fashion, any point of contact to tell the institution's story. Such contacts include patients; visitors; staff; volunteers who are not auxiliary members, but work directly through the institution's department of volunteer services; customers who use the facilities of gift, thrift, and coffee shops; school officials and students who participate in health careers programs; and others with whom the auxiliary may come in contact in the course of its many activities.

The community relations committee could, for instance, consult with the auxiliary's coffee shop committee about the possibility of incorporating into the menus a message explaining how shop profits earned by the auxiliary have been used in recent years to enhance patient care. Or it might suggest to the auxiliary's volunteer services committee that stimulation of the interest of patients in viewing the institution as a community-serving health care center can best be accomplished when they are recovering and not too anxious about themselves. Committee members could help distribute educational materials, such as brochures or leaflets, concerning the institution's services. Members might also provide wheelchair tours of the facilities for convalescing patients.

At the same time, the community relations committee should be actively involved in developing special projects of its own, such as: joining forces with other agencies in the community to seek solutions to the drug problem for local youth; initiating a blood donor program for its institution and encouraging community participation; or helping the institution to provide information on its family planning clinic, with auxilians distributing posters and pamphlets to stores and social service agencies within the community.

The structure of the community relations committee should provide for the public relations functions of the auxiliary. Thus the committee should include one or two individuals who are communications specialists. This particular combination of functions within a single committee permits better coordination of information activities within the auxiliary itself. It also enhances the development of a well-integrated information program between the auxiliary, its institution, and the community.

The public relations functions of this committee involve keeping the local newspapers and radio and television stations aware of the auxiliary's efforts on behalf of its institution. This task can be handled directly by the committee's public relations specialist or through the institution's public relations department, which may prefer that all press releases and correspondence relating to the auxiliary be sent out under the institution's auspices.

Also within the domain of the public relations specialist are such responsibilities as arranging for auxiliary leaders to appear on radio and television programs; conducting a speakers' bureau, using articulate auxilians; creating publications dealing with auxiliary activities, such as a newsletter for its own members; or developing promotional materials for special auxiliary-sponsored events, and planning these affairs.

It is obvious that contradiction, duplication of effort, and misinterpretation can run rampant when too many people are working for the same or related purposes, but in unrelated ways. Therefore, the community relations committee should frequently review its own internal plans and also refer to other committee chairmen for feedback on auxiliary activities.

In addition, the community relations committee should consult regularly with the public relations-community relations department of its institution, to ensure that efforts toward reaching the institution's staff, the public at large, and the media are unified and productive and create a coordinated image of the auxiliary's purpose in relation to both institution and community.

Another example of creating a standing committee to handle a distinct action program concerns activities sponsored by the auxiliary for the institution's employees and professional staff.

Activities such as the provision of hospitality to foreign interns and residents, social events for nursing students and others being trained in the institution, or the planning of the annual party and other special events for employees are all efforts, similar in purpose, undertaken on behalf of the institution. Such activities should be made the responsibility of a specially designated committee.

Legislative action represents still another example of a distinct program that would justify the creation of a standing committee. The range of responsibilities that might be assigned to that committee is described in the AHA publication *Guidelines to Federal Legislative Action for Auxilians* (ref. 5) and in brochures published by many state hospital associations. (Note: If the auxiliary is a separately incorporated organization exempt from federal income taxation, the exemption may be jeopardized if more than a "substantial" part — usually considered five per cent — of its total activities is legislative in nature.)

2. *Give each committee authority to subdivide its responsibility.*
Assignment of a particular task to a subcommittee, a special
task force, or an individual committee member can be a useful
device for spreading the work load while simultaneously maintaining a cohesive action program. Decisions on the necessity of
distributing responsibility should be based upon a realistic appraisal of the tasks to be done. The division of the community
relations-public relations responsibilities into separate functions
of the same committee is a primary example. It illustrates the
need for a close, cohesive relationship within a committee structure and, at the same time, provides a means of relieving the
pressure on any one person or group, permitting more freedom
to concentrate on the particular task required and to exercise
greater creativity in the process.

3. *Use existing committees, whenever possible, to handle new
activities; create new committees only when absolutely necessary.*
Unless there are valid reasons for creating a new committee,
or until any new activity has reached full-committee proportions,
it is advisable to use existing committees to handle new projects
as they arise. As an example, an auxiliary may wish to join
forces with other agencies in the community to sponsor a "Health-
O-Rama," a mobile unit that visits various supermarkets in the
area, dispensing information about preventive health care.

Should the community relations committee expand its sphere
of activity to include work on this project, or does the situation
require the creation of a new committee? The answer lies in the
auxiliary board's evaluation of the responsibility. If the auxiliary's role in the project is a small one, it would be both impractical and unnecessary to organize a new committee immediately.
However, if after a year's trial the auxiliary has committed more
of its resources than originally expected in maintaining its part
in the "Health-O-Rama," establishing a new committee might be
justified.

Conversely, an auxiliary could immediately, and with justification, create a new committee to provide a nutrition improvement
program for the elderly in the area — supplying funds, cooking
skills, and staff for meal stations throughout the community.
This is a specialized service, requiring a special type of volunteer
and a close working relationship with the institution's dietary
staff.

Under most circumstances, the operation of gift and coffee shops should be assigned to separate standing committees, for these are distinct action programs. However, there is little reason to establish a separate gift shop committee to stock and staff a small counter in the coffee shop, which sells candy, greeting cards, and a few drugstore items. This responsibility would logically belong to the coffee shop committee, pending the time when the auxiliary could launch a full-scale gift shop.

When the auxiliary's board is in doubt about creating a committee to handle a new activity, it is suggested that the ultimate purpose of the proposed project be analyzed thoroughly. For instance, an auxiliary may wish to provide aid and comfort to non-English-speaking patients. If this undertaking is conceived as simply supplying foreign language reading materials to these patients, the project should be assigned to the community relations committee. However, if the auxiliary envisions its commitment in a larger sense — that of developing a foreign language phrase book for use by hospital employees who frequently come into contact with non-English-speaking patients or sponsoring a series of foreign language classes for hospital employees — then the auxiliary should create a separate committee for these specific purposes.

4. *Be prepared to change committee structure and/or responsibilities in adapting to changing circumstances.*

The prime example of the need for this particular guideline is the considerable change of circumstances that occurs when a salaried director of volunteers is appointed to the staff of the institution. At the very beginning of this new relationship, a clear, mutual understanding among the administration, the auxiliary, and the director of volunteers as to her specific responsibilities, and a positive attitude among all concerned, will make the transition period easier and more productive. It will also help to establish a firm basis for a warm and friendly collaboration between the director of volunteer services and the auxiliary leadership in the interests of their common goal.

In making its adjustment, the auxiliary should be aware that the establishment of a department of volunteer services within the institution's organizational structure, as well as the appointment of a director, does not diminish or eliminate the auxiliary's commitment to patient care and services — but only the manner in which it carries out this commitment. The auxiliary continues to be a major source of volunteers. However, the role of its volunteer services committee becomes that of a supportive group, supplementing the efforts of the department of volunteer services. Because of its very purpose and nature, the auxiliary is uniquely qualified to provide substantial assistance to the one department of its institution that is most closely allied to the community and to the auxiliary's own essential function.

In the process of transferring its original responsibilities to the new director of the volunteer services department, the auxiliary's volunteer services committee gains new ones: serving as liaison between the director and the auxiliary; serving as a sounding board for the director of volunteer services on policies and operational matters directly affecting volunteers; generating ideas, as they develop within various auxiliary committees, that may be helpful to the director in initiating services for the institution; and assisting the director in recruiting and carrying out other departmental responsibilities that are mutually determined.

There should be no tendency on the auxiliary's part, however, to transfer to the director more responsibilities than she can appropriately and actually assume. An auxiliary might attempt to delegate the task of writing its newsletter, or of scheduling appearances for members of its speakers' bureau, to the director of volunteer services. It may even wish to send the director, as its representative, to meetings and conventions. These activities are clearly within the auxiliary's bailiwick and should not be shunted elsewhere. The auxiliary that depends on the director in matters unrelated to the department of volunteer services will quickly lose purpose, vigor, and membership. The functions and responsibilities of the department of volunteer services are fully described in the American Hospital Association's manual *The Volunteer Services Department in a Health Care Institution* (ref. 11).

When a department of volunteer services is established within an institution, it is essential that the different roles and responsibilities of that department and the auxiliary's volunteer services committee be clearly delineated.

Without well-defined areas of operation, neither the department nor the auxiliary can reasonably expect to perform efficiently or effectively. As a result, confusion, misunderstanding, and disagreements arise, making an already sensitive area more sensitive and projecting the division of responsibilities into a major issue!

Caroline Flanders, former assistant executive director of the United Hospital Fund of New York, clarifies this distinction:

What is needed at all times is a clear definition and mutual working understanding of (1) what a hospital auxiliary is, (2) what a hospital volunteer service department is, (3) what the hospital administrator expects from each, and (4) what each may expect from the other.

The auxiliary and the office of volunteer service or the volunteer service department are not organizationally one and the same thing. They are not identical or interchangeable. They are not in competition; neither usurps the authority or assumes the responsibility of the other. Their basic aim is the same, serving the hospital, but they travel quite different roads toward it.

An auxiliary is a self-governing membership organization, an entity with its own personality, accountable directly to its hospital administrator. Moreover, an auxiliary's concerns today are broad, ranging far beyond volunteer service within the hospital.

A volunteer service program, on the other hand, whether or not it has a salaried director, is responsible to administration for its hospital's inservice volunteer personnel. Volunteers are in fact, and by choice, unpaid, part-time workers; as such they are a significant part of a hospital's total manpower. In today's professionally administered hospital, a director of volunteer services holds an important place in its personnel administration.

An individual may be both a member of the auxiliary and an inservice volunteer, but each role requires quite different things of him (ref. 26).

To create a workable program for implementation of inservice volunteer activities, it is necessary for the department of volunteer services and the auxiliary to mutually develop a precise understanding of this division of responsibilities.

In view of the fact that community involvement is going to be claiming an increasingly greater share of the auxiliary's time and effort, both the auxiliary and the institution must recognize that the inservice program represents a self-contained unit, which is controlled by the institution. This, in turn, permits the auxiliary to fulfill its obligations to the community, while continuing to provide support for the inservice effort.

The following approach to the division of responsibilities is therefore recommended:

- The chief executive should clearly delineate the areas of responsibility of the inservice program. He should provide a job description for the person administratively responsible for this program. The job description should accurately reflect the duties as well as the relationships within the institution and to the auxiliary. This approach is recommended because the department of volunteer services is an institutional department and the director reports to the chief executive, not to the auxiliary.
- The auxiliary should then establish the charge to its volunteer services committee in such a way as to provide the kind of assistance actually needed, without interfering with the responsibilities of the person directing the inservice program for the institution.
- The institution should employ the director of volunteer services. She should be chosen, as should all hospital personnel, according to the job classification of the position, which should specify the qualifications that the institution requires. It is generally recommended that the institution employ someone from outside of the auxiliary as director.

If an auxilian *should* be placed in this position, her selection by the chief executive should be based upon her qualifications for the particular job, not solely upon her past experience as an auxiliary member. In addition, when an auxilian serves as director of volunteer services, her first responsibility is to the institution, and it takes precedence over her relationship to the auxiliary. This parallels the situation that occurs when an auxilian serves on the institution's governing board.

In an institution in which there is no salaried director of volunteer services and the auxiliary provides an individual to fill this position, she should be selected with the approval of the administration. Notwithstanding her ties to the auxiliary, her primary responsibility is to the institution for the direction of its inservice program.

- If the institution has a paid director of volunteer services, it is suggested that the salary be provided directly by the institution. This is necessary because the director is employed *by* the institution, having met its criteria in order to obtain the position. This principle should be applicable regardless of the actual origin of the money — whether it is provided for in the institution's budget, the auxiliary's treasury, or an outside philanthropic source.

The volunteer services committee of an auxiliary functions in a supportive capacity when there is a department of volunteer services within the institution. When there is no such department, however, the volunteer services committee assumes a fuller responsibility and becomes a functional substitute for that department.

Any volunteer activities (inservice programs) conducted within the institution are administered by the committee, and the committee chairman functions, in essence, as the director of volunteer services. The committee is responsible for the recruitment and training of volunteers who, when prepared for their roles, work under the supervision of the institution's professional staff.

For example, if there were a need for volunteers to work in the family planning clinic, assisting in educating and counseling obstetrical patients on the services offered there, then the volunteer services committee would work directly with the medical staff and the administration to develop and implement this program. The committee would supply the volunteers, administer the training program under the auspices of the professional staff, and assume responsibility for the ongoing operation of the program.

Conversely, when the department of volunteer services does exist within an institution, and the volunteer services committee believes there may be a role for volunteers in the family planning clinic, it would suggest this expansion of activities to the director of volunteer services. If approved, the department would assume responsibility for including interested auxilians among the volunteers recruited for this particular program.

Ad Hoc Committees

By definition, an ad hoc committee is short-lived. It is created by the auxiliary's board of directors for a specific and limited task that, for any one of several reasons, may be inappropriate to assign to a standing committee.

An excellent example of the type of task best assigned to an ad hoc committee is a periodic and comprehensive review of the bylaws. This ad hoc committee should be composed of individuals who are knowledgeable and deeply committed to the auxiliary's purpose, yet free from the pressure and demands of daily activities and sufficiently detached from ongoing programs to be as objective as possible.

Well-constructed bylaws that adhere to basic principles should not require constant revision. However, the wise auxiliary will want to be sure that its bylaws are relevant and current, and a review every two to three years by a special committee can satisfy this need. During the period between reviews, the board of directors should be constantly aware of the status of the bylaws and prepared to initiate changes as the situation demands. Under these conditions, there should be no need for a standing bylaws committee. All too frequently, when an auxiliary has such a committee, the bylaws are in a continuous state of flux and are much too detailed.

An ad hoc committee is also particularly suitable when a given task requires the expertise of persons who may not be auxiliary members. For example, in reviewing its scholarship program or other types of financial aid to education, an auxiliary should seek the advice of a representative from the local high school system, such as a guidance counselor; a financial need analysis expert from a college or university; perhaps a high school student; a member of the institution's governing board; and, of course, the institution's attorney. These individuals should be invited to join several auxiliary members (from the appropriate standing committee) on the ad hoc committee, in order to study the situation, make recommendations, and then disband. However, these outside advisers should be able to serve on the standing committee that implements the program, should the auxiliary feel the need to retain their input on a more permanent basis.

Although different in many respects from a standing committee, an ad hoc committee should be fitted into the functional operating structure, with the nature of its assignment determining whether it belongs within the service or the community relations area or whether it relates to the self-maintenance functions of the auxiliary.

Coordination of Committee Activities

Coordination of committee activities is essential to good auxiliary management. This responsibility falls to the president-elect, who works with the several committees involved in the basic, self-maintenance functions, and to the vice presidents for community relations and for service, who coordinate the activities of committees in their respective areas. Such assignments of responsibility encourage teamwork and smoother, more efficient working relationships among all concerned. They are also a vital part of leadership development. Finally, they free the auxiliary president for her role as interpreter of the auxiliary to the institution and the community.

Committees in Action

In order to act effectively, each committee should have responsible leadership and written guidelines that are carefully prepared, faithfully reflecting the real nature of the committee's function.

Leadership

Because the auxiliary entrusts to its committees its major action programs and self-maintenance functions, committee chairmen are key individuals in the leadership group. To a great extent, the auxiliary's success or failure in achieving its goals depends upon their capabilities. Similarly, a chairmanship offers to an individual auxilian the opportunity to demonstrate her potential for other, and perhaps more important, leadership responsibilities.

Each chairman is appointed by the auxiliary's president, with the approval of the executive committee (or the board, if there is no executive committee). Chairmen should be selected on the basis of previous experience, ability to fully understand the committee's responsibilities, ability to work well with others and to motivate them, and perseverance, so that objectives are accomplished. Each chairman should be given as much guidance as she needs from the executive officers, but as little direct supervision as possible.

The chairman has responsibilities *to* her committee as well as accountability *for* its actions. She should fully comprehend the importance of involving members in determining how the committee's objectives should be met, as well as in other committee activities; prepare an agenda for each meeting; report on board actions that affect the committee; and represent the committee's viewpoint (not just her own) at board meetings.

A vice chairman and a secretary complete a standing committee's leadership team. Both are appointed, as are all members of the committee, by the chairman after she confers with the president and seeks suggestions from the membership relations committee. A major test of a chairman's sense of responsibility to her committee, as well as to the auxiliary, is her interest in training the vice chairman for a future leadership post.

The auxiliary president should appoint the chairmen of ad hoc committees with the approval of the executive committee (or the board of directors, if there is no executive committee). Some auxiliaries may prefer to have the chairman of the ad hoc committee exercise the prerogative of selecting committee members. Regardless of whether the auxiliary president or the ad hoc committee chairman makes the final selection of committee members, however, such selection should be made in accordance with the guidelines established by the board of directors for that specific committee.

Guidelines

The guidelines for all standing committees are included in the administrative policies and procedures and, for all ad hoc committees, in the minutes of the auxiliary's board of directors. Guidelines for both standing and ad hoc committees should define the number of persons who will serve on such committees and set a limit of not more than two consecutive years to the tenure of standing committee chairmen. The guidelines should also determine the special qualifications required for membership on a specific ad hoc committee.

The most significant item in the guidelines is the committee's charge — the clear delineation of its responsibilities. This charge should be broadly stated, but never vague. It should specify the committee's objectives, but not how to attain them. It should set standards of performance, but not list the specific duties to be performed. A charge, therefore, is broader and more flexible than a job description, in order to encourage individual initiative.

As an example, the charge to the gift shop committee might read as follows: It shall be the responsibility of the gift shop committee to operate, within the institution, a shop selling gifts, sundries, and other items that may appropriately be stocked in such a shop. The shop shall be operated primarily as a convenience and service to patients, visitors, and staff, in such a manner as to bring credit to the institution and the auxiliary; and, insofar as may be consistent with its primary purpose and special nature, as a means of providing a financial contribution to the institution. The committee shall be expected to exercise good business judgment and follow standard good business practices in managing the shop.

Next in importance to the committee's charge is a delineation of relationships — to members of the institution's staff or to other auxiliary committees. As an illustration, the public relations section of the community relations committee is responsible for clearing its activities, including the issuing of press releases, with the institution's public relations director (or, in certain instances, with the administration). This requirement should be noted in the committee's guidelines.

The guidelines should also describe the number of members constituting a quorum for the transaction of business. In addition, they should cover certain matters of procedure: that parliamentary rules are followed, that accurate attendance records are kept, and that minutes of each meeting are prepared and filed with the auxiliary's recording secretary.

Finally, the guidelines should indicate that utilizing the planning and evaluation processes, as they relate to the committee's own performance, is a part of the committee's responsibilities. For a detailed analysis of this subject, see Chapter 11, "Planning and Evaluation."

chapter 6
Legal Considerations

There is an increasing concern of auxiliaries about their legal rights, responsibilities, and duties. For the hospital, too, the volunteer poses certain legal problems. Indeed, all individuals participating in these activities are interested in whether there are any legal pitfalls which may ensnare them in their work.

Mrs. Newton B. Millham,
former chairman,
Committee on Volunteers,
American Hospital Association

Legal Status of the Auxiliary

Logic dictates that those responsible for establishing the legal status of an auxiliary should always confer with the institution's attorney and follow his advice. He should explain that, in legal form, an auxiliary can be organized as (1) an integral part of its parent institution, (2) an independent corporation, or (3) an unincorporated association.

Generally speaking, unless the legal considerations in a local situation suggest otherwise, it is preferable that the auxiliary be organized as an integral part of its parent institution. In most instances, this is the legal form that, from the standpoint of tax liability and the availability of liability insurance coverage, provides maximum benefits to the auxiliary and its members. It also gives the institution ultimate control over the auxiliary's activities on its behalf.

If the auxiliary is organized as an independent corporation, the institution is deprived of exercising direct authority over the auxiliary. This arrangement can create problems regarding the auxiliary's accountability to its institution and can also destroy the sense of unified purpose that is so essential in the auxiliary-institution relationship.

Of the three alternatives, the auxiliary as an unincorporated association is the least desirable. For example, if a member of such an auxiliary commits an act that injures a patient or a visitor, there is the possibility that all the other auxiliary members will be considered legally responsible. There may also be difficulty for the auxiliary in obtaining liability insurance coverage. In the area of taxation, revenue obtained from gift shops and other auxiliary activities may not be exempt from federal taxes.

When the auxiliary is organized as an integral part of its institution, certain procedures should be followed:

1. The bylaws of the parent corporation should be amended to specifically authorize the establishment of the auxiliary, or a resolution of the institution's governing board should authorize or approve the organization of the auxiliary (see Appendix B).

2. The auxiliary's bylaws should be approved by the institution's governing board and should include a provision to the effect that the auxiliary is an integral part of the parent corporation and that the auxiliary's bylaws cannot be amended without the consent of the governing board.

3. The authority to establish bank accounts for the auxiliary should be broadly delegated to the auxiliary, or the types of accounts should be specifically described. In either case, the institution's governing board should authorize the action by a resolution.

4. The auxiliary should periodically file financial reports with its institution, and these reports should be included in the annual financial statement and all federal and state income tax reports of the parent corporation.

5. If the auxiliary is soliciting gifts in its own name, rather than in the name of the institution, it should request the

chief executive or the institution's attorney to file appropriate forms with the Internal Revenue Service to receive a determination that any such contributions will be deductible to the donor. (If the institution itself is tax-exempt, it may be simpler and equally sufficient to request that gifts be made directly to the institution.)

6. If it is contemplated that the auxiliary will engage in business transactions under its own name (such as contracts to purchase merchandise for a gift shop), a certificate of doing business under an assumed name should be filed by the institution with the appropriate legal agency, if required by state law.

Liability

Auxiliary-Operated Shops

Shops operated by an auxiliary are, to a limited extent, commercial ventures in that they employ business methods for their success. As such, they are subject to federal laws and regulations; to state laws that vary among the states; and, in some instances, to local ordinances. Consequently, there are some specific legal implications for the auxiliary.

Assuming that a hospital or other health care institution has qualified for exemption from income tax, and that the auxiliary is organized legally as an integral part of such an institution, then the income derived from the sale of shop items generally would not be subject to federal income tax. According to the Internal Revenue Service, gift shops, coffee shops, and other businesses operated exclusively for the use of the hospital are not "unrelated trade or business," and therefore the income from such enterprises, used for charitable purposes, is not taxable.

The Internal Revenue Code would normally impose a tax on such a business if it were not substantially related to the charitable purpose. An example of an unrelated purpose might be a hospital coffee shop operated primarily for profit, rather than to make its services conveniently available to those within the institution. On the other hand, a coffee shop operating to fulfill a charitable purpose would primarily serve ambulatory patients, professional staff, general employees, and visitors.

State sales taxes might or might not apply to the purchase of items in shops. There is a considerable variety among these laws, and it is quite possible that a tax might apply to one type of merchandise and not to another, or might be assessed in one state and not in another. There are also use and excise taxes that, under certain circumstances, would not apply, but it is advisable to verify this.

Two categories of concern pertain to liability in auxiliary-operated shops: injuries, either to other volunteers or to customers, caused by a negligent volunteer while working in the shop; and injuries sustained by a volunteer herself. The problem of liability, when it is associated with any type of volunteer activity, is discussed in detail in the AHA manual *The Volunteer Services Department in a Health Care Institution* (ref. 11). Another AHA publication, *Auxiliary Gift and Coffee Shop Management* (ref. 1), includes a checklist for legal and business considerations related to gift and coffee shops.

In the case of thrift shops operated by auxiliaries, *separately incorporated thrift shops* may qualify for exemption from federal income tax on earnings if substantially all of the merchandise sold there is donated or if substantially all of the work is performed by volunteers. If thrift shops are operated by *separately incorporated auxiliaries,* the taxable status is still open to question and must be resolved on an individual basis.

To ensure correct understanding of legal matters related to auxiliary-operated shops, as well as any other legal matters, it is advisable for auxilians to consult with their institution's attorney. He can provide the most current interpretation of the laws as they relate to the operation of auxiliaries, with specific application to the individual auxiliary involved.

Other Areas

Two other aspects of liability that should be considered are (1) automobile liability insurance for auxilians when driving on institution-related or auxiliary-related business and (2) liability insurance for special events sponsored by the auxiliary but held outside of the institution.

Regarding automobile insurance liability, an auxilian who drives her own car on institution or auxiliary business must generally assume financial responsibility in the event of an accident. Therefore, adequate personal insurance is a necessity at the outset. Should the auxilian be driving an automobile owned by the institution, however, any liability she may incur should be covered by the institution's insurance. Toward this end, it is helpful for the auxiliary president to consult with the institution's attorney to ascertain whether the institution's general automobile liability coverage contains a provision for the use of its vehicles, for business purposes, by volunteers and auxilians.

When the auxiliary conducts a special event away from the institution's premises, "special events" liability insurance coverage should be obtained. This special coverage will protect the auxiliary from claims filed (1) by the general public in case of personal injury or (2) by the ownership of the place where the event is held in case of property damage. This coverage should include:

- "Premises-operations" coverage for the site of the event.
- "Products" coverage, if any food or beverage is served.
- "Dram shop" coverage, if liquor is served. State laws should be checked for the extent of the coverage required.
- "Incidental contractual" coverage, if the premises are leased by contract and if the contract contains a "hold harmless" agreement.

The auxiliary president should consult the institution's attorney concerning the limits of liability required and the necessity of including "dram shop" and "incidental contractual" coverage. The types of insurance discussed here can be purchased either by the institution as a supplement to its basic insurance policy or by the auxiliary directly. Such coverage should be easy to secure and relatively inexpensive, because it can be obtained for only the term of the specific event.

Income Tax Deductions for Auxilians

Certain expenses incurred by auxilians and other volunteers on behalf of their institutions qualify as federal income tax deductions — only when volunteers are not reimbursed and when such deductions are itemized on the appropriate Internal Revenue Service form. These expenditures include:

- **Transportation expenses.** For driving their personal automobiles, whether locally or otherwise, on institution or auxiliary business, auxilians may deduct whatever is allowable. In-town taxicab trips relating to business are also deductible for the amount expended. When out-of-town travel costs (plane, train, bus, or taxicab) are borne by auxiliary members, they may deduct their actual expenses.

- **Business trips.** Cost of meals, hotel or motel lodging, or other related personal expenses may be deductible when a person travels as an official representative of the auxiliary or institution. This would include the cost of attending conventions or educational meetings, such as registration fees and so forth. Regarding individuals who attend such meetings in an unofficial capacity, however, personal expenses are *not* deductible. The only deductions permitted are costs incurred for the benefit of the auxiliary, such as the purchase of educational publications.

- **Uniforms.** The expense of purchasing and maintaining uniforms or similar clothing appropriate only for volunteer service on behalf of the institution may be deductible.

- **Donations of merchandise.** The cash value of merchandise donated to auxiliary-operated shops may result in a tax deduction — providing that the shop devotes all of its profits to charitable purposes. However, the cost of items purchased in auxiliary-operated shops is not deductible by the customer.

- **Contributions of money.** Funds donated to the auxiliary or its institution are deductible. In like manner, dues are deductible to the extent they exceed membership benefits and thus constitute a contribution. Included in this category would be the cost of purchasing tickets to special events sponsored by the auxiliary, such as fund-raising dinners or theater benefits. However, the portion of the cost that is actually deductible is the amount remaining after subtracting the price of the dinner, theater ticket, or whatever basic service has been provided.

The above information is furnished primarily to alert auxilians to the fact that certain federal income tax deductions may be available to them. The allowance of such deductions may vary from time to time, or additional deductions may be available in certain cases. Deductions on state income tax also may be allowable. Auxilians should obtain professional consultation before submitting these deductions on an income tax return.

Scholarships and Fellowship Grants

Because of the need for qualified personnel to fill positions in the rapidly expanding health care field, many auxiliaries are already earmarking specific portions of their contributions budgets for scholarships and fellowship grants in health careers. A detailed presentation on the development and implementation of these and other forms of aid to education is given in the American Hospital Association's manual *Financial Aid Programs in Support of Health Occupations: A Guide for Auxiliaries* (ref. 3).

As with any type of financial aid program conducted by an auxiliary, various legal and tax implications are involved, and these are the primary concern here. Of foremost importance to the auxiliary in the proper handling of its specific scholarship and fellowship programs, whether ongoing or in the formative stage, is the maintenance of close and continuing contact with the institution's attorney. As stated earlier, he should be the primary source for information on tax and other laws affecting the individual auxiliary.

The most important aspect of an auxiliary's commitment to a scholarship program is the effect of the program on its institution's tax-exempt status. The Tax Reform Act of 1969 redefines the standards that tax-exempt organizations must meet if they are to retain this status, and not be reclassified as private foundations. It is necessary that the auxiliary do nothing to jeopardize the tax-exempt status of its institution.

To ensure the continuance of this status, the auxiliary should consider the following basic guidelines in designing its educational awards programs:

- The class of individuals who are eligible to compete for scholarships or fellowships should be large enough to encompass a cross section of society, rather than limited to those already involved with the institution — such as junior volunteers, children of volunteers, and hospital employees or their children. The number of awards given to this latter group should not be disproportionate, in order that the selection of recipients remains nondiscriminatory.
- Any person seriously interested in pursuing a health career should be invited to apply. The applications for these awards should be broadly distributed through community service

organizations, religious groups, high school career counselors, and so on.

- Recipients should be selected on a merit basis including such criteria as prior academic performance, achievement on aptitude and ability tests in the health field, career interest demonstrated by past volunteer activities and work in the health field, financial need, and motivation as determined by personal interviews of applicants.
- Certain categories of applicants should be considered ineligible for awards. These include individuals related by blood or marriage to members of the selection committee, or those related to substantial donors to the scholarship fund. The selection committee should include outside parties as members.

From the recipient's viewpoint, there are possible tax obligations upon acceptance of a scholarship grant. The auxiliary should be aware of the conditions attached to such financial grants when it designs its educational awards programs.

According to the Internal Revenue Service, a student receiving financial aid for education is exempt from paying federal income taxes on his award provided that he is not pursuing his studies or research for the benefit of the grantor; that he is not compensated for past, present, or future services; and finally that he is not, through his studies, merely qualifying himself for an advanced position with increased compensation.

chapter 7
Fund Raising

Can auxiliaries afford to use 1960 standards for
fund raising and spending when the rules of the '70s and '80s
are different? Our present programs may seem
adequate, but let us have the courage to measure them
against current hospital and community needs.

Mrs. Newton Millham,
former chairman,
Committee on Volunteers,
American Hospital Association

Traditional Role

Fund raising was originally the auxiliary's reason
for being. This primary function evolved naturally, in response
to the position hospitals occupied in society before the advent of
modern surgery and medical technology.

Begun as almshouses for the care of the poor before the Middle
Ages, hospitals — until the mid-1700s — provided little more
than charitable shelter and lodging for the indigent, the pilgrims,
the wayfarers, the sick orphans, the homeless, the incurably ill,
and the insane. When severe epidemics erupted over the cen-
turies, hospitals were used on occasion to house the sick, but the
death rates were so staggering, because of unhygienic conditions
and lack of medical knowledge, that they became places of last
resort. As depositories for the poor, hospitals were shunned by
physicians, who recommended that their private patients be

cared for at home. This situation was exemplified by New York City's Bellevue Hospital, which, in the early 1800s, housed 2,000 paupers with perhaps 200 sick persons among them.

Caring for the sick in terms of nursing and medical services was an incidental outgrowth of caring for the poor and destitute. By the mid-1700s, the emphasis slowly began to shift toward concern for actually treating the ill, but even these patients were still in the charity class. To help hospitals subsidize the cost of caring for these individuals, the forerunners of today's auxiliaries came into existence.

In 1752 a group of wealthy widows and single women of Philadelphia contributed funds to Pennsylvania Hospital (the first general hospital in the United States) for drugs shipped from London for indigent patients. Additional groups, in other hospitals, eventually formed to provide money, food, and clothing for the hospitalized poor and to perform the first service-oriented activities of sewing and rolling bandages. These fledgling efforts were the genesis of the hospital auxiliary, although it was not until 1863 that the first formally organized auxiliary appeared on the American hospital scene. The introduction of the auxiliary as a charitable organization, concerned primarily with helping the poor, also marked the first of several stages of development through which auxiliaries were to pass.

With anesthesia coming into use by 1850 and aseptic techniques for the prevention of infection emerging around 1865, successful surgery became a possibility. Hospitals gradually became places where physicians could send their acutely ill patients — those who could afford to pay — for care and even cure. Although the stigma attached to hospitals was disappearing, health care was still an expensive privilege, and the poor had to rely upon the beneficence of the groups of wealthy women comprising hospital auxiliaries.

By 1941, auxiliaries were still helping to support charity patients, but the major thrust of fund-raising projects had broadened to include a larger portion of hospitals' operating expenses. Money for new buildings or renovations, room furnishings, and medical equipment now claimed priority in fund-raising programs.

When World War II erupted, auxiliaries were offered a unique opportunity to demonstrate their true ability to provide patient care as well as money for their institutions. With the induction of health care personnel into military service, the need for volunteer manpower was acute. Auxiliaries responded superbly, expanding into new areas of service that brought them into direct and regular contact with patients and supplementing the work of regular nursing and related staff, thus freeing the professionals to concentrate on the medical aspects of their work. *Most important, however, they contributed a more personalized kind of care and attention, which made the hospital seem less like an institution.*

This integration into hospital services marked the second stage of auxiliary development, adding the dimension of direct service to the traditional fund-raising role. It also signified the beginning of community consciousness on the part of auxiliaries, as they began to recognize their function as a link between their institutions and the community at large. After the war, auxiliaries stayed on in health care institutions, not to substitute for paid personnel but to continue to provide the supplemental services that contribute to total patient care.

New Role

Since then, auxiliaries have traveled a great distance both conceptually and functionally. As the institutions they represent have been evolving into providers of comprehensive health care services to the total community, the services offered by auxiliaries have been changing and expanding accordingly. As hospitals have been shifting away from being isolated entities and into their appropriate role as community institutions, auxiliaries have been finding new interpretations of service to their communities in terms of dollars and effort.

This emphasis on "community" is expressing itself in another way: a continuing trend toward increased cooperation among hospitals in the coordinated delivery of health care to their communities. Exemplified by such concepts as shared services, this cooperative approach is a response to the need to use health care dollars more economically and effectively. Reflecting this trend, auxiliaries within the same community are giving serious thought to combining their fund-raising efforts for specific programs and projects. This results in better utilization of auxiliaries' human resources and merging of financial resources for more immediate realization of necessary programs and projects.

Although money is, of course, still needed by health care institutions, emphasis on subsidizing operating expenses has generally diminished. A large portion of these basic costs is now covered by patient revenue and third-party payers (private health insurance and federal and local governmental funding). Monies that once were expended for medical care of the indigent, or for building funds and equipment purchases, may no longer be specifically required for these purposes. Many institutions also have their own development departments, which conduct extensive fund-raising campaigns, at both community and corporate levels, and apply for government grants.

What this means for auxiliaries is a challenge in a third stage of auxiliary development. As the financial demands of health care institutions are refocusing to accommodate newly emerging needs, so must the fund-raising concepts of auxiliaries be rethought: the role of fund raising in the auxiliary's total program, the types of activities to be conducted, and the projects into which money will be channeled.

If auxiliaries wish to respond in a contemporary and meaningful way to their institutions' financial needs, they should consider regearing their programming so that fund raising is represented by a diversity of community-oriented activities in addition to the traditional annual cycle of social events, bazaars, and similar projects.

Today's fund raising is defined in relation to two primary objectives: as a by-product of direct service-oriented activities that are conducted on the premises of the institution, and as indirect service-related projects that are generally conducted in the community and are a means of promoting interaction between the institution and the community. In both types of fund raising, consultation with and approval by the institution's chief executive are essential.

Fund Raising as a By-Product of Service

Auxiliary fund raising that is an immediate by-product of direct service-oriented activities derives earnings from the operation of enterprises within the institution. Such enterprises are established to provide service to patients, personnel, and visitors on a permanent, year-round basis. Gift shops, coffee shops, gift carts, and television rental services are primary activities in this category.

Criteria for this type of fund raising are:

- Provision of service should always take precedence over making profits.
- The opportunity to provide educational information about the institution, both to the volunteers who staff such operations and to the consumers of these services, should be utilized by the auxiliary. For example, the gift shop could distribute an informational flyer with every item purchased, or the coffee shop could display posters designed to tell the institution's story. Menus could carry inserts on the achievements of the auxiliary and the institution and could describe the ways coffee shop earnings are used.
- To be truly successful, an enterprise should be acceptable to the community it serves. As an illustration, the gift shop should carry merchandise that reflects the wants and needs of the patient population and visitors, not the desires of the auxiliary's members, which may be quite different.
- Efficient operation, utilizing sound business practices, should be a primary objective in the functioning of these on-the-premises shops and services. Such enterprises should be managed with the same care and skill that would be invested in a regular, profit-oriented business.

Fund Raising as a Community Relations Function

If an auxiliary undertakes additional fund-raising activities, beyond the direct service-oriented type, they should serve as vehicles for promoting better interaction between the institution and the community. Viewed in this manner, fund raising becomes an extension of an auxiliary's community relations function. Responsibility for conducting community-oriented fund-raising activities should therefore be assigned to a fund-raising committee that is either a subcommittee of the community relations committee or, at the least, closely interrelated.

Interaction is rooted in good communication between the two entities: the institution and the community. Ideally, the institution seeks to learn what the community wants and needs in new or expanded health care services and attempts to meet these needs, but it must derive a portion of the initial funds from the community in order to do so. Conversely, the community, being well informed about the institution's current programs, philosophy, and projected plans, understands the reasons that money is being requested and how it will be expended. This dialog builds mutual trust and engenders active community support for the institution.

Fund raising of this type encompasses activities of an indirect service nature that are generally conducted in the community rather than within the confines of the institution. In addition to encouraging community support, these activities bring in funds for demonstrable needs within the institution's program and serve to educate the public about the functions and goals of the institution and the auxiliary. Again, as with service-oriented projects, participating auxilians are exposed to an educational process about their institution.

Activities in this category include such permanent, year-round projects as thrift shops and memorial funds. Shorter-term, more concerted efforts are the annual fund-raising campaign conducted by the institution with the auxiliary's assistance; sponsorship of sporting and cultural events; presentation of annual bazaars, rummage sales, or other merchandise offerings; special money collection days; and any other regularly scheduled activities that offer opportunities to reach a broad spectrum of the public and augment its knowledge of the institution.

Criteria for this type of fund raising are:
- The project should enhance the community's concept of the institution as a dignified and respected facility for health care. In order to reflect this image most favorably, an auxiliary should be highly selective in the types of fund-raising activities it sponsors.
- As in service-oriented fund-raising projects, the community's acceptability is an important factor in the choice and operation of an indirect service project — but in a more comprehensive and significant way. An auxiliary wishing to reach all strata of the community should know its composition, leaders, and past responses to various types of fund-raising efforts, if a successful venture is to be undertaken.
- The project should not compete with the fund-raising activities of other community-based organizations in relation to

timing and type of activity. Good communication with out-side groups and coordination of plans can prevent wasteful duplication of effort in which everyone loses.

- Those who contribute to fund-raising projects should gen-erally receive something of value in return. For special events such as art exhibits, symphony concerts, or theater perfor-mances, for example, the programs could contain a general acknowledgment to the contributors who have made the benefit possible through their purchase of tickets. Events such as fairs or bazaars, which provide activities, merchan-dise, and food, give supporters something for their money.

- Those who give to fund-raising campaigns should receive letters of appreciation and information on the uses to which the funds are applied. Another method of expressing grati-tude for financial support is by thanking the community as a whole, perhaps via an advertisement in the local news-paper. Both procedures can be handled either by the auxiliary directly or by the institution's development department.

Assessment of Fund-Raising Programs

A progressive auxiliary should recognize the need to frequently review its fund-raising program in terms of goals, methods, and relevance of such activities to the auxiliary's total program. At this point, the fund-raising committee enters the picture, to assume its appropriate responsibility for this impor-tant function. Having responsibility for an aspect of community relations (and thus a committee within the province of the vice president for community relations), the fund-raising committee will require some well-considered responses to the following questions:

- Does the current fund-raising program meet the criteria discussed in the previous sections?

- Are the uses for funds contemporary and relevant in view of today's health care needs? These uses are exemplified by community-oriented projects such as public education pro-grams on preventive care, medical research programs, out-patient care and freestanding neighborhood health clinic programs, and financial aid to support health careers for new entrants into the field and to supply continuing educational opportunities for present employees of the health care institution.

- Is the auxiliary still delegating funds exclusively for new equipment, for offsetting operating deficits, and for renovation and repair? If so, shouldn't funds contributed by the auxiliary be used for the expansion or initiation of programs for which the institution can obtain no other types of financing?
- For the auxiliary whose institution is not currently receiving adequate funding from third-party payers for operating expenses, it may be essential to contribute funds for these purposes. If so, is the auxiliary buying equipment that is not really necessary but simply desirable to have or that unnecessarily duplicates specialized equipment already available in the area?
- Is an enormous or disproportionate amount of effort being spent on fund raising that yields a relatively small return or that has been contributing a steadily decreasing percentage of the institution's funds for special projects or operating income? If so, are such projects also monopolizing the time and interest of members to the detriment of other auxiliary programs, which could make better use of volunteer manpower?
- If the institution has its own development department, could more be accomplished if the auxiliary cooperated with that department and participated in an overall fund-raising plan?
- Are present fund-raising efforts really contributing to the institution's ability to better provide health care services to patients and the community?
- Are such efforts helping to establish or augment a responsive relationship of goodwill between the institution and the community? Is community education a major goal in the conducting of fund-raising programs?
- Is the auxiliary's educational program giving members the informational tools they need to *be* effective fund raisers?

Fund Raising in Action

Today's fund raising, through the media of indirect service-related projects — our main concern here — should be a well-defined process, operating in relationship to established criteria and following certain patterns in planning, education, and evaluation. Using the standards for current fund-raising programs discussed in the previous section, for example, an auxiliary has a contemporary frame of reference for determining the eligibility of projects and their goals from the beginning. If it is then decided that a project deserves implementation, the following approach is suggested.*

Planning

Planning is the businesslike approach. Prior to the actual initiation of a fund-raising effort, the auxiliary should present its ideas on potentially valuable uses for such funds to the institution's chief executive. In some instances, the administration may present the auxiliary with a list of its primary needs. Whatever the situation, mutual consultation should result in agreement on the institution's most urgent or important programs and services for which the auxiliary will provide funding.

At this point, the auxiliary can develop a detailed, written plan of operation for achieving each major objective. This plan should include establishing the projects that will carry it to completion and describing how these projects will function; designating the leadership and the organizational structure required; checking the legal aspects of the venture with the institution's attorney; designing a publicity campaign; and outlining a financial plan, containing an estimate of fixed advance costs and gross income.

The timing of special fund-raising campaigns and events in relation to other community projects is important, as mentioned earlier. In addition to avoiding duplication in the type of event, projects also should be limited to a reasonable number each year and should be well spaced so that the community's welcome is not worn thin, nor its support for the auxiliary's parent institution eroded.

It is important, at the outset, that the auxiliary plan to keep accurate records of all income and expenditures for each project, in addition to an estimate of the amount of effort required and a detailed description of the types of effort expended. This pro-

*This section and the balance of the chapter deal specifically with fund-raising projects of an indirect service nature. The subject of direct service-oriented fund raising is handled extensively in the American Hospital Association publication entitled *Auxiliary Gift and Coffee Shop Management* (ref. 1).

cedure is essential if the results of a project are to be evaluated realistically. It also provides persuasive data for community education programs and supports the auxiliary's requests for funds in the next project.

Education

Successful fund raising depends on education. Communicating the facts during a fund-raising campaign or in the conducting of a specific project is an educational process that affects not only potential contributors through the community but also auxiliary members. To be convincing representatives of their cause, presenting their case authentically to the community, auxilians need all the supportive information on the project and their institution that they can obtain.

This need for information is particularly significant in view of public concern about hospital costs and general resistance to fund-raising appeals generated by the increasing number of campaigns conducted by numerous organizations within the same community.

Informing the Auxiliary

An effective educational program for auxilians should be developed cooperatively by the fund-raising and the membership education committees. It should be designed to cover every possible aspect of the current fund-raising project and should go beyond the immediate objectives and introduce additional information about the institution. In this manner, larger issues concerning the institution often can be related to requests to fund special projects.

For example, if a continuing education program for hospital employees is the objective of a fund-raising project, details about the program's benefits can serve as a springboard for a discussion of the institution's responsibilities toward its employees. This discussion can lead logically to presentation of a broader issue: the institution's concern for the improvement of the quality of patient care.

The program of education for auxiliary members should include complete information about the objectives of the project, with a clear description of the service or program to be subsidized, the equipment or furnishings to be purchased, or the improvement to be financed. The detailed, written plan of operation, developed by the auxiliary prior to the initiation of the project, can serve as a basic orientation piece.

In addition, auxilians should be provided with the vital statis-:ics concerning their institution's operating expenses; utilization)f funds raised through the auxiliary's efforts; the number of .ndividuals who benefit from various services offered by the institution; and any other relevant information. This thorough background exercise can help them in dealing with every reaction, ranging from general curiosity to hostile criticism, as they encounter their personal associates and the general public. This type of information also should be used as general educational material for auxilians. (See the section entitled "Membership Education" in Chapter 8, "Education.")

Although much of this information may be found in the institution's annual report, it would be beneficial for the auxiliary to conduct some in-depth research, consulting with the appropriate departments of its institution for current facts.

The types of questions auxilians should be prepared to answer encompass the following areas of concern:

- Why, specifically, does this health care institution need more money? Will all the funds collected be used for a particular purpose? When and how will the contributor see evidence of the funds expended? How much of an income tax deduction can the contributor expect to take for his donation?

- How many persons in the community received health care services last year or in recent years from the institution, and what was the total amount of money expended by the institution to provide these services? Categorizing the patients who used these services, how many were admitted for inpatient care, the emergency department, or the outpatient clinic? What was the cost to the institution in each of these areas?

- Were the benefits to patients primarily in the improvement or expansion of basic health care services, or were there no appreciable changes in the delivery of these services? Did the institution attempt to reach out into the community to provide innovative health care and health education programs?

- How much money did the institution actually realize from the auxiliary's operation of the gift and coffee shops during the past year?
- What were the total operating expenses in the institution's last fiscal year? How much was spent on salaries or wages, and how much paid to suppliers, including costs of food, pharmaceuticals, utilities, and so forth? The often controversial topic of a health care institution's financial needs takes on a new interpretation when these needs are related to the financial support of actual individuals and essential services.

Informing the Community

Education for the community should be an integral part of any fund-raising effort — for the total group in general and for the project's supporters in particular. Fund raising that doesn't generate in-depth information about the sponsoring institution at the same time that the request for financial support is made is likely to meet resistance or eventual failure in achieving its goals. Here, the fund-raising and community relations committees would join forces to create a community education program.

The problem inherent in fund-raising appeals, particularly in communities that have been overly saturated with campaigns, is the credibility gap that has developed between the expression of an institution's financial needs and the public's ability to believe.

Caroline Flanders, former assistant executive director, United Hospital Fund of New York, clarified the situation when she stated: "Hospitals are costly; but let us remember that hospitals do not hoard money. They pour it right out again into their communities. Try to visualize what would happen . . . if all the hospitals — voluntary or governmental, local, state, and federal — didn't write any checks for one month for either employees or suppliers. . . . Hospitals are, first of all, institutions for healing persons and promoting community health; but obviously, they contribute importantly to their communities' economic health as well" (ref. 27).

A carefully planned information program helps to close the community's credibility gap, while acknowledging that potential contributors are intelligent individuals who, when approached for money, deserve more than a superficial explanation for the appeal. They should also be made to feel that as community representatives, their financial and moral support for their own community institution is necessary to the success of the project.

As the medium for the transmission of this vital information to the community, auxiliary members are providing more than a one-shot educational program. They are establishing the groundwork for future fund raising and thereby building mutual trust with each successive effort.

The information program for contributors doesn't end with the completion of the fund-raising project. To make the public aware of the health care value of its donations — facts to which it is entitled — and, more important in the long view, to sustain active interest in and support for the institution's programs, follow-up activity on the results of the project is essential.

This can take the form of a letter to contributors, sent out some time after the basic letter of acknowledgment, offering current information on the amount of money raised and progress in realizing the project. A newsletter, issued annually or biannually, can provide a running commentary on the specific project to which they contributed, in addition to a more general discussion of the institution's programs. Such follow-up promotes a positive image of the integrity of both the auxiliary and the institution. Auxiliary members, of course, should also be kept informed of the outcome of all fund-raising efforts.

To ensure effective fund raising, auxiliaries should recognize that it is a "people process" — that personal visits by thoroughly oriented auxilians to individuals and organizations within the community can do more to establish rapport, augment the educational procedure, and gain continuing support than any number of mailings. Specially prepared promotional material for distribution to potential contributors and an ongoing publicity campaign are part of the educational package.

Evaluation

Realistic evaluation is an essential process that must be accomplished if fund raising is to be a meaningful and productive part of the auxiliary's program. The possibility that it may also be an arduous, time-consuming process should be balanced against the future rewards of having progressive and successful fund raising.

Two major questions should be posed at the completion of a fund-raising project: Were the profits worth the time, effort, and money invested? Did the project help the institution and community to interact on a positive level? If the responses are negative, the project should be analyzed, with further examination along these lines:

- Was the type of project the wrong choice? Or was the error in the planning or the educational program?

- Is it possible to improve upon the present project or campaign, or should the auxiliary's total approach to fund raising be reviewed?

- Has a certain type of project outlived its usefulness or validity to the community?

- Was the appropriate manpower available for the project, in terms of leadership and membership? Were the individuals who conducted the project capable of functioning effectively in the particular circumstances involved?

- Can the community be better educated concerning the work of the institution in ways other than through fund-raising projects?

- Could a major portion of the time and effort expended by the auxiliary on a fund-raising project of this type be more productively invested in other kinds of fund-raising activities, or even on projects not related to earning money but beneficial in other ways to patients and the institution?

On the basis of questions such as these, the auxiliary should analyze each fund-raising project honestly and make decisions for the future that will promote the best interests of the institution and the community it serves.

Assigning Responsibility

It is generally most practical to delegate the responsibility for the management of fund raising to the auxiliary's finance committee, with a subcommittee designated specifically for fund raising. Working in concert with the community relations committee for the actual conducting of the project, and with the finance committee for the management of the budgeting procedures, the fund-raising committee can operate successfully.

Uses for the Auxiliary's Funds

With health care institutions receiving an increasing share of financing for patient care, buildings, and equipment through private health insurance and government sources, the auxiliary, in conjunction with the institution, must seek important new ways to use its philanthropic dollars. The first step is for the auxiliary to become fully cognizant of the health care needs of its community — not only as they currently exist, but as they are likely to be within the next five to ten years.

Then, after careful study, the auxiliary should develop some well-conceived and clearly defined suggestions for redirecting its funds in ways that will fulfill these needs through the 1970s and into the following decade. In presenting these ideas to the administration, a progressive auxiliary can be the catalyst for a whole new way of viewing the auxiliary's role by the institution and, eventually, the community.

The possibilities for future-oriented programs and services are numerous, and they will expand as the auxiliary continues to assume broader responsibilities on behalf of its institution's delivery of health care.

The auxiliary should be aware of the differing financial obligations inherent in short-term versus long-term funding of programs, regardless of the duration of the programs themselves. Short-term funding, lasting perhaps a year or two, requires an initial financial commitment, generally involving a moderate amount of money. Such funding can be used as seed money to launch a program, with the institution soon assuming the expense of maintaining it, or to provide a brief period of support for an ongoing program. Long-term funding, on the other hand, requires a financial commitment to a program over a period of years. Whether financial commitments are short-term or long-term, however, the decision to fund programs will affect an auxiliary's contributions budget. Such a decision, therefore, should be carefully considered, to ensure that the amount pledged will be available each year.

Some suggested uses of auxiliary funds are:
- Supporting educational programs for employees, ranging from purchasing on-the-job training manuals and equipment to providing scholarships, stipends, or tuition refunds for continuing education, or financing a total continuing educa-

tion program or department, or a portion thereof. This type of commitment to employee education offers opportunities for career mobility in that many employees can advance beyond the mere improvement of existing skills; rather, they can move into totally new areas of the health care field that offer greater professional rewards.

- Helping to recruit health manpower by sponsoring a health careers day at the institution and inviting the community, or providing speakers and exhibits at high school career promotion events. Funds can also be diverted into the production and distribution of health careers literature for use in school libraries, hospital waiting rooms, and physicians' offices, and by high school counselors. Scholarship, stipend, and tuition refund programs can make health careers more attractive to those in the community who are financially disadvantaged. For information on designing financial assistance programs for employee education or new careers in health care, auxiliaries should refer to the American Hospital Association publication *Financial Aid Programs in Support of Health Occupations — A Guide for Auxiliaries* (ref. 3).

- Financing and establishing day care nursery services that can reduce absenteeism of employees caused by child care responsibilities, permit the return to employment of individuals who had left the institution's work force to care for small children, and enable employees to return to work following maternity leave.

- Funding research and experimentation programs, ranging from establishing a health sciences library for staff use to financing a specific research project.

- Arranging to compile, print, and distribute a directory of health care resources within the community and updating it on a regular basis.

- Funding a library for patients on the premises of the institution.

- Participating in the funding of community-oriented health services in the institution's outpatient clinic or in freestanding "satellite" clinics operated by the institution and devoted to community health care. Within this type of ongoing project, trained auxilians could participate in such activities as menu planning for patients on special diets; nutritional counseling of patients under the direction of the institution's dietitian; engaging in discussions on budgeting, family planning, new-baby care, and other family-related subjects, and distributing appropriate educational materials in conjunction with these discussions; and assisting outpatients in completing their admitting forms. Auxiliary funds could also be directed into building and/or decorating and furnishing outpatient or community health clinics if other funding is not available.

- Initiating educational programs for the community on preventive health care and the management of chronic illness. Such programs, which could be conducted at the institution or out in the community, would offer facilities for disease detection and immunization in addition to educational opportunities. Seminars, "clinics" on particular problems, health fairs, and mobile educational units are among the media that could be utilized for the dissemination of information. (For a more detailed description of community education programs, see Chapter 8, "Education.")
- Initiating a program, in cooperation with appropriate community organizations, to provide temporary foster care for abandoned or abused children.
- Cooperating with the social services department of the institution to provide funds for food, clothing, baby-sitting services, and any additional necessities for needy patients when they leave the institution.
- Helping the institution recruit volunteers for its inservice volunteer department from a broad spectrum of the community. By offering to subsidize transportation, uniforms, and meals, the auxiliary can help attract a representative corps from among the disadvantaged, older persons living on fixed incomes, and others who would not be able to serve unless financial assistance were provided.
- Providing funds for community health projects, in cooperation with other local groups such as mental health associations, visiting nurse organizations, private social welfare agencies, and other auxiliaries. When the institution recognizes the need for establishing and/or maintaining certain programs and services within the community, the pooling of

financial resources can be a most advantageous method of
securing the necessary funding. It is often a more immediate
way of raising money and getting the program in operation,
compared to such efforts, on an individual basis, by institutions or agencies. Mutual funding can be applied to health
career scholarship programs; halfway houses for mentally
ill persons, drug addicts, or alcoholics; well-baby clinics; or
educational programs on preventive health care.

- Contributing a portion of the funds to help establish a home
  care program for its institution and participating in the
  program by visiting convalescing patients in their homes,
  providing transportation for patients to rehabilitative treatment facilities, and so forth. In this manner, the auxilian
  becomes a functioning member of the home care team.
- Financing a mobile blood procurement program.
- Establishing a "health hot line," that is, a telephone information and assistance service operated by auxilians under
  the supervision of professional staff. The service could provide help in emergency situations such as treatment for
  poisoning, drug overdoses, suicide attempts, and related
  problems. In addition, it could guide members of the community to appropriate health care resources for more general, nonemergency problems. In bilingual communities,
  auxiliaries should attempt to recruit volunteers with appropriate language skills to operate this type of information
  service. It should be emphasized that any volunteers participating in a "health hot line" will require in-depth training to
  properly handle the emergency situations and to learn correct referral techniques for health care services.
- Developing a language phrase book and accompanying educational program for auxilians, inservice volunteers, and
  staff in dealing with non-English-speaking patients.

The Institution's Fund-Raising Campaign

In an institution that has a development department with professional fund raisers conducting capital fund
drives or long-range development programs, an auxiliary may be
requested to engage in activities in an assisting capacity. In
complying with such a request, the auxiliary is fulfilling a basic
purpose of service to the institution.

To work successfully in tandem with the parent institution requires that the auxiliary adopt a somewhat different attitude and approach to its fund-raising role. In this type of situation, the auxiliary's fund-raising activity is conducted under the direction of the institution rather than under its own aegis.

However the auxiliary participates, its activities should be made an integral part of the overall fund-raising plan. This means that in some instances, the auxiliary may have to relinquish traditional fund-raising projects because they would conflict with the master plan; in other cases, auxiliary-sponsored projects can be incorporated into the master plan.

If the auxiliary is to be involved at all in a major fund-raising campaign of its institution, it should be involved from the beginning, with the auxiliary's representatives appointed to the overall planning group. To ensure their integration into the campaign and successful participation, auxilians should receive an in-depth orientation on their specific responsibilities. Provision should also be made for evaluating the auxiliary's efforts when the campaign is completed.

It is through the recognition of this mutuality of interest and the need to maintain a high information and communications level that the institution and the auxiliary can work together productively in this situation.

chapter 8
Education

. . . changes in the world of hospitals urgently
call for auxiliaries to go beyond the traditional involvement
and programs. . . . The auxiliary must come to an
understanding of, first, its own hospital and community
needs and, second, the forces bringing change
to the hospital world — locally, regionally,
and nationally.

William P. Moore,
administrator,
South Davis Community Hospital,
Bountiful, Utah

The auxiliary that fulfills its dual obligations of membership education and community education with imagination, diligence, and conviction helps to ensure its institution's ultimate success in meeting health care needs.

Membership Education

A high level of membership commitment exists in the auxiliary that provides a communicative and comprehensive educational program. Conversely, when the quality of the program is poor or when it has no priority in the auxiliary's concept of membership relations, members are less motivated and therefore less committed to the goals of the auxiliary.

As one of the auxiliary's primary obligations to its members, an ongoing educational program — the responsibility of the membership education committee — has the greatest significance to the involvement process. When provided on a continuing basis, such a program is capable of stimulating and reinforcing membership commitment and sustaining active interest. (See Chapter 3, "Membership and Leadership," under "Obligations to Members.")

This constant educational effort is indispensable to the achievement of the auxiliary's goals, particularly when it encompasses the important facets of the national health care picture, the sweeping changes occurring within it, and their relevance to the auxiliary's own institution. Only a membership aware of the broader implications of its work will be prepared to underwrite a dynamic program of auxiliary service and to provide the leadership to meet the changing needs of its institution and community.

From the outset, the total approach of the membership education committee toward fulfilling its responsibility can be an important factor in determining whether the membership is a well-informed, cohesive, and productive group; a group of apathetic and uninvolved individuals; or something in between, a kind of semimotivated, not quite committed group. Beginning with orientation sessions for new members and periodic reorientation programs for the general membership, continuing into creative programming for regular membership meetings and special intra-auxiliary workshops, and extending outward to membership participation in local, regional, and national educational seminars and conferences, the membership education committee can provide the impetus for a vital and enduring learning experience.

Restricting educational opportunities to the auxiliary's officers and committee chairmen contradicts the basic principles of leadership development advocated earlier in this manual. (See Chapter 3, "Membership and Leadership.") Consequently, to implement the educational process, the membership education committee should actively promote firsthand participation for all members.

Orientation

A member's first in-depth educational exposure within an auxiliary occurs at the time of orientation. This introductory process should establish a precedent for all the educational efforts that will eventually follow; presentations should be well structured and comprehensive and should instill the urge to participate actively. Because orientation is, in a sense, preparation for future involvement, it should create a lasting first impression, indicating that the auxiliary is vitally interested in its members and recognizes the need for thoroughly educating them.

New auxilians should obtain a wide-angle view of the auxiliary's basic and particular functions and its relationship to the institution; the institution's physical plant, staff, and the services offered through its various departments; and the relationship of the auxiliary and the institution to the community, in terms of meeting current and future health needs. In addition, new members should be made aware of the importance of maintaining good relations with the broad spectrum of individuals encountered by auxilians. To accomplish this kind of comprehensive education, a number of persons representing the auxiliary, the institution, and other community organizations will need to contribute to the orientation program.

Auxiliary personnel who should be directly involved in this introductory process should be selected by the membership education committee. For example, the president, as the chief liaison officer between the auxiliary and the administration of the institution, could be enlisted to clarify the relationship that exists between the two entities. To obtain a comprehensive view of the two major areas of the auxiliary's activities, the vice presidents in charge of service and community relations would be the appropriate choices.

Representing the institution, participants in the auxiliary's orientation program should include such individuals as the chief executive or one of his assistants from the administrative department or the director of public relations-community relations. They should be able to provide a total picture of the institution, including internal functions and relationship to the community.

The actual process of orientation begins with the provision of materials for auxilians to review. Foremost among these are the auxiliary's bylaws, which should receive a particularly thorough perusal if new members are to understand organizational structure and become aware of their rights and responsibilities. Information on the auxiliary's history and record of service to the institution is also important. Basic background material describing the history of the institution, current and long-range plans for the provision of health care, departmental organization, and operating procedures can be furnished by the administration.

To implement understanding of the relationship of auxiliary committees to the total institution, organizational charts would be most helpful. Correlation of functions exists in certain areas such as the community relations committee of the auxiliary and the institution's public relations-community relations department, the auxiliary's finance committee and treasurer and its counterpart in the institution's comptroller, the coffee shop committee and the institution's dietetic department, and the volunteer services committee of the auxiliary and the department of volunteer services of the institution. Close working relationships between these related operations can create a mutuality of purpose in support of the institution's objectives.

For firsthand exposure of new members to the physical plant and operations of the institution, an orientation tour should be conducted, with commentary provided by the auxiliary leader and appropriate personnel within the departments.

All these methods of education can incorporate visual aids such as flip charts, films, slide presentations, tape recordings, and even videotape presentations when a closed-circuit television operation is available at the institution.

If the auxiliary is truly seeking to establish a membership that is broadly representative of the community, it will be composed of individuals from all social, economic, and educational backgrounds. Therefore, the methods of orientation should be designed to make many different kinds of people feel comfortable with the group. Informality in approach is one way to create a relaxed atmosphere. Conducting orientation sessions during a meal or over coffee, rather than in classroom style, is an excellent technique in this direction.

Auxilians who lead these discussions should attempt to establish an atmosphere of friendly openness and directness, encouraging comments and questions while reducing fear of criticism. New members should, ideally, gain confidence during the orientation process. They should be made to feel that their potential contributions are already considered valuable by the auxiliary and the institution and that they will be accepted as an integral part of the institution's family through their membership and service in the auxiliary. Simultaneously, leadership should convey the expectation that new members will be required to maintain high standards of performance and that they will be assisted by the auxiliary and the institution in meeting these standards.

It is better not to assume that an elementary orientation to auxiliary and institution functions is too basic. Even the sophisticated volunteer, experienced in other health care settings, needs to know the particulars of *this* situation.

A successful orientation program also shows concern for the needs and interests of the individual auxilian. Each member is unique in what she can offer in skills and experience. In addition to group orientation sessions and a tour of the institution, individual meetings should be held between the chairman or members of the membership relations committee and each new auxilian. These personal discussions should determine how the particular abilities of the new member can best be utilized and at the same time satisfy her individual needs and expressed interests.

If an orientation program has been communicative, stimulating, and cognizant of the importance of auxilians as individuals, the resulting enthusiasm and productivity of the new members will bear testimony to its effectiveness.

Reorientation

The procedure of orientation should not be limited to new members, but should apply to all auxilians, regardless of length of membership. Periodic reorientation programs are an effective technique for maintaining members' interest in the auxiliary's work, updating their knowledge of the institution, and demonstrating that the auxiliary values its members enough to keep them well informed. Within the framework of membership meetings, for example, department heads from the institution and appropriate auxiliary members can provide information on new or changing functions. Tours of other health and educational institutions within the community, including local colleges involved in cooperative teaching programs, can be beneficial to auxilians.

The reorientation process is particularly essential for the auxiliary whose educational programs for members have been allowed to dissipate or become somewhat archaic in approach and method. Or, if an auxiliary is being reorganized, redefinition of its structure and operations may be required and this can be accomplished via a reorientation program. Whatever the situation, reorientation efforts should be a continuing part of the auxiliary's educational program.

Membership Meetings

Membership meetings offer a prime opportunity for education. By providing interesting and truly informative programs, several purposes are served: the members' understanding of functions of the auxiliary and the institution and their relationship to the community is enhanced, and attendance at meetings is stimulated.

The membership education committee assumes the responsibility for designing programs that attract and maintain the interest of the group. If subject matter is germane to auxilians and is presented imaginatively and in depth without being too long, members will be motivated to invest their attention. The more incisive and comprehensive the presentation, the more it compliments the collective intelligence of the group and heightens the group's feelings of value.

One suggestion for a program would be the functions of the auxiliary in various areas of service and a corresponding evaluation of effectiveness. To obtain a broad viewpoint, the auxiliary's programs could be compared to those of other auxiliaries, both locally and nationally, detailing similarities and differences in approach to the same situations. The president of another auxiliary, or a representative from the state hospital association, could be invited to address the group and provide valuable assistance in the evaluation process. (See Chapter 11, "Planning and Evaluation.")

Generally speaking, auxiliary programs should be tailored to the individual situation — the particular hospital the auxiliary serves, the community in which the auxiliary exists, and the auxiliary itself. Given this general framework, *The Volunteer Leader,* which is published by the American Hospital Association, is a useful source of program ideas. Almost every issue includes an article whose subject could be developed into an interesting and informative program for an auxiliary meeting.

Other subjects of interest could encompass improvements that could be initiated to help auxilians function more effectively within the institution and the community; the nature of the

auxiliary's current relationship to other community organizations and methods of expanding it, including increasing opportunities for communication; and the emerging community needs
in the health care field and how the auxiliary can help its institution to meet them. Speakers from other community organizations
could be requested to present profiles of their groups' functions
and their viewpoints on the institution's accomplishments in
meeting health care needs, while suggesting possible cooperative
ventures between other community groups and the auxiliary.

A periodic procedure for membership meetings could be the
inclusion of a department head or staff member, who could brief
the membership on current concerns. Similarly, when new or
specialized programs and services are inaugurated by the institution, the appropriate staff member should be requested to
present relevant information. In addition to keeping auxilians
up to date on the institution's operations, this educational technique establishes rapport between the institution and the auxiliary and helps to implement good working relationships between
the two entities. As such, it should be an integral part of any
ongoing educational program.

Seminars and Workshops

The membership education committee can also conduct
intra-auxiliary educational seminars dealing with more comprehensive topics, such as the legislative process and how the auxiliary can opt for better health care legislation, both locally and
nationally; the projected expansion program of its institution in
both services and physical facilities and how it relates to auxiliary activities; and the vastly changing health care scene with
emerging new forms of care. This last topic could explore hospital mergers, which require cooperative efforts between two or
more auxiliaries; or the emergence of new health care delivery
systems via health care corporations and health maintenance
organizations, which may call for changes in the concept of
volunteer services.

Another subject that would provide interesting educational
possibilities for a seminar or workshop is the sensitive area of
human relations, including the influence of interpersonal communication on the relating process. Because auxilians come into
contact with many publics — the community at large, the insti-

tution's employees, patients, and other volunteers — this subject is basic to the creation and maintenance of effective communication. To supply the basic orientation, professional staff members from the institution's departments of social service or psychiatry could be enlisted to present their views. Community resources could also be utilized, by inviting other local organizations, such as health and welfare agencies, to contribute their expertise on this subject and on the psychology of the sick. Nearby universities can provide faculty from their sociology or psychology departments to participate in lecture and discussion groups. In this manner, both the academic and social service segments of the community can contribute substantially to the education of auxilians.

Other Educational Opportunities

Educational goals can be furthered by the attendance of representatives from the general auxiliary membership, as well as officers and committee chairmen, at the various conferences, workshops, and institutes presented throughout the year by district, state, regional, and national hospital associations, and local health and welfare agencies or civic groups. Such meetings can be invaluable in helping to broaden the horizons of auxiliary members. Attendance at inter-auxiliary workshops can also be helpful in implementing understanding of the auxiliary's functions and problems and in exploring possibilities for new roles.

Adult education courses offered by local colleges and schools are a resource that can help provide a broader background of knowledge for auxilians. Subjects such as organization management, communications, leadership training, interpersonal relations, budgeting, and health education are all relevant to auxilians for the purpose of program development and for dealing with the auxiliary's daily problems.

In addition, members' involvement in the work of regional planning committees relating to the health care field, or board or committee membership in other community agencies with similar goals, should be encouraged.

Another type of educational activity for auxilians, although nonparticipatory in nature, is exposure to the various media offerings concerning health care and related matters. As one of its responsibilities, the membership education committee should alert auxilians to the availability of this information via television and radio programs, magazine and newspaper articles, hospital publications, tapes, and films.

Library Resources

The auxiliary that believes in reaching out for education to the various types of organizations just discussed will be on the receiving end for the educational newsletters, journals, manuals, pamphlets, and bulletins produced by these local and national groups. Publications from these outside sources as well as the auxiliary's own records, reports, and related materials belong in a central location where the entire membership can make use of them. Too frequently, the auxiliary's president and other officers are the only individuals who are exposed to these publications and reports.

It is the responsibility of the membership education committee to provide a reference library service for the auxiliary to ensure that the total membership has a continuing opportunity for education. To achieve this purpose, a small section of the institution's library should be utilized. However, if this is not possible, the committee should secure some other suitable office space within the institution. A committee member can be assigned to review all incoming informational materials from outside sources and bring relevant facts to the attention of the total board or individual board members. When information gleaned through this process is deemed significant to the general membership, it can be presented by officers or committee chairmen at membership meetings or via the auxiliary's newsletter, which is produced by the membership education committee.

Responsibility for organizing the auxiliary's records and reports within the library resides with the auxiliary's recording secretary. She should maintain this collection of information in a chronological, well-organized manner, and ensure that it is accessible to membership. Regarding the retention of minutes from board meetings, specifically, the secretary may want to index them by subject matter, as well as by month and year, for quicker access.

The ability to easily retrieve all such information is extremely important to the auxiliary, because this material is used in the preparation of annual reports, for planning and evaluation procedures, and for maintaining continuity from one leadership group to the next. (See Chapter 10, "Records and Reports.")

Supplementary Materials

Auxilians should be provided with yearly fact sheets or an information kit containing material on the financial aspects of its institution's operations and vital statistics on services furnished to the community, information on the auxiliary's financial contributions, and other such matters. The information supplied to auxilians engaged in fund-raising activities is appropriate for general use on a year-round basis. (See the section entitled "Education" in Chapter 7, "Fund Raising.")

An auxiliary newsletter can be utilized as a major educational vehicle, presenting information on broad aspects of health care in addition to the standard items about the auxiliary and the institution. Every issue should include at least one article on a major health problem and its implications for health care institutions. Such articles could cover environmental problems, the need for blood donations, the difficulties of refuse disposal in the community, problems in dealing with third-party payers, drug and alcohol abuse, pending legislation that would affect health care institutions and the quality of care, and feature stories on the community's health care needs and the ways in which they are being met by other community health organizations in addition to the auxiliary's own institution.

In the event that the auxiliary doesn't publish its own newsletter, it should use its channel of communications with the public relations-community relations department of its institution. By providing the type of information described above to this department, for possible inclusion in the institution's newsletters for contributors and the general community, the educational process for auxilians is maintained on a continuing basis.

To ensure that auxiliary members have the opportunity for exposure to educational publications in general, and those of the American Hospital Association in particular, the auxiliary should subscribe to additional copies of *The Volunteer Leader* for all or at least some members of the board, should receive additional copies of *Washington Developments* for selected members, and should purchase additional manuals for specific committees. *The*

Volunteer Leader, in particular, is a valuable tool for every auxiliary member. To encourage its use, one individual could be assigned responsibility for soliciting subscriptions. This person should promote the idea of each auxiliary member having a subscription to *The Volunteer Leader,* as it is a publication specifically geared to the concerns of auxilians and directors of volunteer services and it is available at a nominal cost. Other AHA publications could also be ordered via this individual. For a selected list of AHA publications, see Appendix B, "The American Hospital Association as a Resource."

Community Education

The Obligation to Inform

Like membership education, community education is a basic obligation of auxiliaries, and it is an intrinsic part of the auxiliary's community relations function. Cohesive, well-organized community education programs are a necessity, because they are capable of:

- Motivating moral and financial support for the institution by providing information on its programs, services, and effectiveness in meeting the community's health care needs.
- Providing the community with access to informed opinion on the larger issues affecting the delivery of health care, which should be of primary importance to every consumer.
- Helping to orient the community on preventive health care, bringing the educational process to a personal level.
- Offering the institution an opportunity to obtain community feedback on attitudes toward local health care delivery.

The first capability, which is detailed in Chapter 7, "Fund Raising," is a way of giving something to the community in exchange for its endorsement of the institution. In this regard, pertinent information accompanies the request for support, is provided on an ongoing basis during the realization of a project, and should be a continuing part of all the auxiliary's fund-raising efforts.

In order to facilitate the community's understanding of its problems and needs in the delivery of health care within its immediate environment, it must see these needs in the broader context of the city, state, and national situations. Community attention should be focused upon the key aspects of health care delivery, which encompass access to services; availability versus maldistribution of facilities; fragmentation and duplication of services; and the quality, continuity, and comprehensiveness of health care. The American Hospital Association and the appropriate state hospital association can furnish auxiliaries with pertinent materials and references needed to develop a community orientation on these subjects.

In addition, the auxiliary should make the community aware of each citizen's prerogative to work for better legislation in the areas of health, housing, and the combating of poverty, so that people suffering from environmentally induced illness, for example, will not have to return to the conditions that precipitated their problems. Institutions serving economically depressed communities have long recognized the correlation between medical problems and poor sanitation, inadequate nutrition, improper housing, insufficient heating and ventilation, and the myriad of related conditions that flourish in such environments. Efforts to remedy the situation, in many instances, have been inadequate. However, with community support firmly behind a cohesive program for legislative change, this complex problem may see resolution.

Orientation of the community, through educational programs on preventive health care, is an expression of the institution's concern for the health and welfare of those it serves. As a vehicle for conducting these programs, the auxiliary has the opportunity to reach out and connect with a large cross section of individuals, often in a personalized way. Whether this educational process is carried out on the institution's premises, in a community center or other facility, or via a mobile health care exhibit, the desired results are the same: an informed community, cognizant of the importance of health care knowledge in general health maintenance, aware of the institution's genuine concern for its well-being, and supportive of the institution's present programs and future plans.

A successful educational program also increases communication between the institution and the community, stimulating feedback from the community on its opinions of current health care delivery — its wants and needs, both fulfilled and unfulfilled. Such feedback makes health care provision by the institution a two-way proposition, capable of being defined by both the provider and the user. It also makes responsiveness a real possibility in the relationship between institution and community.

The Auxilian as Educator

As a vital link between institution and community, the auxiliary member has a dual responsibility. To the public, the auxilian frequently *is* the institution. Therefore, she serves as a community relations ambassador, charged with creating and maintaining goodwill toward the entity she represents. More important, she is an immediate and influential vehicle for educating the community in regard to the institution and its role in the health care scene. Her ability to convincingly communicate this story to the public will depend, to a great extent, on how successful her own educational experience concerning institution and auxiliary has been.

A concern for the community's opinion of the institution is an integral part of the auxilian's responsibilities. What the community thinks about the institution can affect its response to fund-raising campaigns, can influence attendance at auxiliary-sponsored fund-raising events, can stifle or enhance the recruitment of individuals into the auxiliary or volunteers into the institution's inservice program, can be a factor in the institution's retention of employees, can determine interest and participation in preventive health care programs, and can affect the status of communications between the institution and the community.

Because all these activities touch on the auxiliary in some way, the individual member is obliged to exert her most persuasive efforts toward interpreting the institution to the community in a knowledgeable, positive manner. Through her relationships with patients, visitors, representatives of other community organizations, the media, and the general public, she can generate the basic information and approach to the community that will elicit understanding and support.

Methods of Reaching the Community

Community education, like membership education, is a continuing process, permeating all levels and types of auxiliary activities. Responsibility for the total community education program should be assigned to the community relations committee, which should then delegate subcommittees to handle specific aspects of this function.

Community education can be defined by the type of approach used to disseminate information about the institution and the auxiliary. The direct approach is represented by events and programs that offer an immediate and overt opportunity to discuss these subjects via personal appearances, verbal presentations, and printed and display materials. Less direct, more subtle techniques include programs that primarily provide service and secondarily offer information.

Whatever the approach, auxilians should learn how, when, and how much to promote the institution and the auxiliary and should be certain that their presentations of facts are accurate and that their interpretations of programs and operations are consistent. A well-conceived and conducted membership education program helps to ensure these conditions.

Direct

Direct approaches to educating the community include:

- Sponsoring and participating in an open house at the institution, with a guided tour of the facilities, followed by a social hour and refreshments.
- Conducting a children's day at the institution, specifically geared to familiarizing youngsters and their parents with facilities and procedures and alleviating the fears that children often associate with hospitals.
- Providing articulate individuals from the auxiliary's speakers' bureau for appearances before other community organizations and professional clubs, to interpret the work of the institution and the auxiliary.
- Organizing and financing exhibits on the institution's services and the factors affecting the costs of hospitalization, for display in the lobby of the institution, in local banks and office buildings, and in the windows of department stores.
- Organizing and financing exhibits on health careers, with specific emphasis on the institution's use of health care personnel, for displays in schools and other appropriate locations throughout the community. Along similar lines, the auxiliary could conduct a "Careers Day" at the institution to stimulate participation in the health professions, or could

arrange and conduct a health careers presentation at local high schools, enlisting the assistance of appropriate staff from the institution.

- Arranging for appearances of auxilians on local radio and television interview and talk shows, to tell the institution-auxiliary story. Newspaper interviews are another excellent method of focusing public attention on the institution, and well-informed auxilians can be available for or even seek out such opportunities. These arrangements with the media should be made through the institution's public relations-community relations department, if it exists, or through the administration.

- Inviting other community organizations to establish liaison or group memberships in the auxiliary, as a method of promoting an educational exchange. The information such members carry back to their organizations and the community can provide a broad base of support for the institution's programs.

- Sponsoring and organizing an annual educational series to be held at the institution or another local facility. The series would be geared to creating community awareness of current changes and advances in medical science and health care delivery, exploring social issues of public concern, and providing information on available health care resources. Programs would be presented by local professionals from the various fields involved. This type of endeavor offers the auxiliary a direct opportunity to simultaneously interpret and promote the institution, particularly if the institution is conducting programs in the areas under discussion. It also brings the most informed opinion from within the community *to* the community in a concerted effort. Subjects could include such concerns as the problems of aging and child development, accident prevention and treatment, and assessing the need for psychiatric treatment and for techniques used in therapy. Another possibility for subject matter would be an in-depth view of a new treatment center at the institution, such as a rehabilitation facility, with the relating of carefully prepared case histories on families dealing with long-term health problems. Each series, whether dealing with a single subject or an assortment, could be presented over a period of months, with one session offered monthly.

- Presenting a "Health Day" at the institution, in conjunction with the auxiliary's annual meeting. The one-day event could offer brief seminars on selected health and social issues and, in addition, could focus on the auxiliary's most successful accomplishments during the past year. Members of the institution's governing board, the chief executive, the medical staff, and other health care professionals from the community could be invited to participate in the seminar programs, as both speakers and audience.

Indirect

Propagating information to the community on a more subtle level — as in the performance of a service, which carries with it the opportunity for education as a secondary aspect — represents the indirect method of education. Every service offered by the auxiliary should therefore be recognized for its intrinsic educational potential, and utilized to the fullest in this respect. Community health education and patient education programs are examples of services that fulfill these requirements.

Community health education programs developed by the auxiliary in cooperation with the institution's medical staff and presented in layman's language to the community help to orient the public, so that it regards the institution as a vital part of the total community health care picture and the auxiliary as a necessary adjunct to that role. Such programs may emphasize preventive health care or may offer information on the ancillary management of certain chronic illnesses.

The format for the presentation of these programs includes seminars, workshops, or "clinics" that could be conducted at the institution, in a neighborhood health care center, or in another community facility. Mobile health care exhibits are also an effective method of disseminating information, such as the "Health-O-Rama" mentioned in Chapter 5, "Committees." These exhibits travel throughout the community, visiting supermarkets, shopping centers, and other points of public gathering.

Still another expression of the institution's concern for the health and welfare of people would be the operation of a mobile medical service in nearby rural areas. A van, containing all the essential equipment for basic medical tests, staffed by the institution, with auxilians serving as contacts and receptionists, could visit medically underserved areas. Physical checkups could be given and information on preventive health care could be distributed.

Undertaking the presentation of a "Health Fair" would be another community-serving possibility for the auxiliary. However, it is recommended that such endeavors be conducted within the context of a state, county, or city fair, or as part of a joint effort with the local council of community agencies or a similar group. A Health Fair would offer a roundup of the most common and current concerns in disease prevention and the management of chronic illness. In addition to displays on these subjects, the fair would feature screening programs, with appropriate detection facilities, for such medical problems as tuberculosis, hypertension, sickle cell anemia, and impaired vision. Immunization for childhood diseases could also be provided on a mass basis.

Subjects in the preventive health care category could cover information for expectant parents on prenatal care, preparation for childbirth, and child care; proper nutrition; personal and household hygiene; health rules to protect against hypertension and heart disease; poison prevention and emergency treatment for poisoning of various types (including lead poisoning); maintenance of mental health; breaking the smoking, alcohol, drug, and obesity habits; and venereal disease.

Educational programs on the management of chronic illness could offer supplementary information on diet, weight control, exercise, and other subjects related to living with an illness more comfortably. Heart disease, ulcers, diabetes, hypertension, sickle cell anemia, arthritis, allergies, and migraine headaches could all be covered.

Patient education programs offer opportunities to the auxiliary to initiate special projects for the benefit of patients, while providing a positive and well-informed viewpoint of the institution's services and exemplifying attitudes toward those it serves. The fact that the institution cares enough about its patient population to provide educational programs for convalescing individuals says much about these attitudes. Because patients are part of the community at large, the first-person impression they carry back to their families, neighbors, and friends can be either a valuable community relations tool or a detriment.

A service the auxiliary could offer in this area would be the purchase and management of closed-circuit television facilities with the studio on the premises. Programs could focus on the posthospital management of chronic illness, with instructions on special diets, physical activity, and so forth. More general programs on principles of personal and household hygiene, proper nutrition, and sound health practices for the prevention of disease would be appropriate subjects for experientially deprived individuals. Auxilians, assuming the role of producers, could develop these programs under the direction of the medical staff and members of the institution's staff who are responsible for patient education. They could also provide personnel for the telecasts, including knowledgeable auxiliary members as well as physicians and related health care professionals. This television system could also be used to permit patients to view their children, when the youngsters are under minimum visiting age.

Another service would be the provision of seed money to enable the institution to establish an identifiable patient education program.

chapter 9
The Dynamics of Meetings

Meetings are held for the purpose of moving the
organization forward. By helping the auxiliary accomplish
its purpose as an organization, meetings, in
themselves, provide a service.

Dorothy Balfanz Teas,
consultant,
formerly staff associate for volunteer services,
Illinois Hospital Association

This chapter concerns the conduct of meetings, not their content, which is covered in Chapter 8, "Education," under "Membership Education."

Psychological Principles

Meetings can fulfill a variety of constructive needs — if they are permitted to do so. This achievement may require both leadership and membership to reconsider their traditional concepts about meetings and to supplant them with some newer approaches. Although meetings will always be vehicles for transacting business, planning, solving problems, and carrying out the basic functions of any group, they are, in a contemporary sense, really much more than any of these.

According to experts in business and group management, psychological motivation, and leadership development, meetings can serve comprehensive and meaningful purposes — whether in corporate or volunteer organizational structures. Meetings should be viewed as opportunities to educate and learn, to be heard and seen by others, to enjoy oneself — thus offering ego gratification and fulfilling social needs — and to develop an organizational team capable of accomplishment as a group; as valuable tools for developing proficient techniques in problem solving, training, and in-depth planning; as motivators of activity; and as steps in the process of developing leadership from within the group. Meetings should be "idea factories," where the best efforts of disparate minds are able to unite in final, productive decisions.

If the auxiliary could conceive of its meetings as offering such opportunities, which are capable of moving the organization forward, it could make meetings more dynamic and effective.

The following sections discuss some of the specific psychological principles underlying the dynamics of meetings in general.

Member-Centered Meetings

Creative and effective meetings are, ideally, member-centered, with members actively participating in the processes of planning, defining, and deciding. Without the permissive atmosphere that encourages this role for members, meetings generally fail to engender the positive attitudes and productivity that ultimately make the auxiliary's programs successful.

Recognition of the importance of each member's contribution to the auxiliary is most apparent during the open forum that meetings should provide. During the give-and-take of discussions, and the eventual decisions to which they lead, members can easily determine whether their input is receiving serious consideration by leadership or only lip service. Members cannot be expected to implement decisions over which they've had no control or influence. If they feel that the board makes all decisions and then expects them to act as a rubber stamp, they will believe that they've been personally shortchanged. This attitude creates resentment, which, in turn, influences the membership dropout rate.

Communicating — Not Just Talking

"The great enemy of communication is the illusion of its existence" (ref. 17). Because such a premium is placed today on successful "communication," the term is often overused and the practice of real communication misunderstood and under-utilized. Certain barriers to effective communication exist; overcoming these obstacles is a primary obligation of any group, through the joint effort of leadership and membership.

Of utmost importance is the maintenance of frankness and honesty within a group — an openness that permits the candid offering of ideas and the airing of disagreement, in addition to fostering a readiness to examine the real problems affecting the auxiliary. None of this is possible when there is a fear of leadership's censure.

If handled correctly the actual encouragement of dissent, popularly known as "creative conflict," can be particularly effective in making progress within a group situation. When discussion and appraisal of new ideas are openly sought, the stimulus for dissent is an inherent part of the process. Meetings provide opportunities for creative thinking and disagreement — leading to other alternatives. This whole cycle of suggestion-dissent-alternative stimulates productive decision making.

Leadership's Role

Two major factors determine whether meetings accomplish their stated objectives: the ability of leadership to use certain techniques in planning and conducting meetings, and the overall attitudes of members toward the auxiliary's operational methods, programming, and leadership.

Shaping the appropriate attitudes of members, in its more extreme forms, smacks of manipulation. However, it *is* the obligation of leadership to attempt to influence membership in ways conducive to the positive functioning of the auxiliary and to motivate members into sharing some of the responsibilities traditionally associated with leadership. Following this route makes membership participation a fact and responsibility for the auxiliary a mutuality.

According to Strauss and Strauss, "We now know (and research continues to emphasize) that participation, and only participation, will release the untapped supply of energy and ideas. Industries have discovered that it results in greater production, cuts down on absenteeism, and provides a real incentive to better the product, whatever it may be. In any organization or group, the situation is comparable. When the members are allowed to build with those at the top, the whole enterprise picks up new energy. It makes little difference whether one talks in terms of man-hours or mind-hours. The salvaging of time and energy is the same" (ref. 55).

In generating new ways of thinking about the roles of leadership and membership in relation to meetings, auxiliary officers and committee chairmen may have to relinquish some of their long-cherished ideas regarding the conducting of meetings and the allocation of responsibility. The chairman who believes that any group is only as effective as its leader may have an ego problem, or, equally possible, may have been bred on the assumption that the authoritarian leader achieves the best results.

Such thinking, and there is evidence that it exists, creates situations in which leaders "habitually, albeit unwillingly, discourage creativity and free speculation," the very essence of productive meetings and membership. The leader "is likely to use her power unwisely. Her influence can transcend the meeting. It is accepted practice for her to exercise this power, and for other members to play to it. The consequence is that her prejudices can inhibit the open proposals of alternatives and new ideas. . . . If only her own ideas get special treatment (and she's developed a sensitive ear to responses that support her own preconceived notions), the result will be boredom, impatience, and more subtly — hostility and rivalry" (ref. 46).

Psychological and sociological research has indicated that the nondirective approach to group work and action is often more successful in creating a mutually supportive type of relationship between leadership and membership than the traditional authoritarian method of operation. Assuming a nondirective attitude requires that the leader cease playing the role of boss and instead begin acting as stimulator and guide.

A leader who conceives of her role in these terms can then envision sharing certain leadership functions and responsibilities with the membership — functions that can possibly be performed better for the sharing. "Though a few superior individuals may be better in their judgment ability, the average of group judgment is superior to most individual judgments. When a problem involves a number of people, group thinking will produce better results than the thinking of any one person" (ref. 55).

Functions to be shared by leadership and membership are:

- Creating and maintaining a permissive atmosphere that encourages open discussion.
- Establishing the group's goals in relation to specific problems, whether the group be board of directors, committee, or general membership.
- Giving serious consideration to all viewpoints expressed.
- Focusing the group's efforts on a solution to the particular problems being explored.
- Summarizing the discussion when it has become confused and needs clarification, has reached a stalemate, or has been overly productive in a short time and requires interpretation.
- Determining methods of improving the group's activities during meetings.

This process of shared responsibility means that in the conducting of meetings, the leader is also a participant in a very real sense. She is not attending the meeting solely to confirm her own opinions, but rather to stimulate and motivate creative thinking, and to help the group translate concepts into action.

Three techniques that may be helpful to leadership and membership in accomplishing these goals are:

- Giving thoroughly descriptive advance notice of meetings, particularly if the business portion will occupy an important place. Along with the agenda for the meeting, a highly informative explanation of the issues to be discussed and resolved should be included. This stimulates thinking in advance and helps to define goals for each meeting. Without the strong frame of reference such materials provide, it is difficult to involve membership mentally, which is the first step toward promoting attendance.
- Utilizing the question as a method of opening up discussion and exploring ideas. Facts, points made in discussion, and suggestions are turned into questions by the leader, who submits them, in a general way, to the whole group rather than to an individual. Questions asked of the leader are then redirected to the group, thereby encouraging participation. "The leader can even use these questions to the whole group to move the meeting along to a new phase of discussion, or to create any other necessary activity. When the need for a summary becomes clear, he can give that, too, in the form of a question, which invites members to comment on any

parts of it they believe inadequate" (ref. 55). The opening questions can be planned by the leader in advance, in order to ensure that the meeting starts on solid ground. The types of questions such an approach generates could include: What is the situation right now? What are the central facts? Is there anything else that should be included? Do you mean _____? What can this committee do about the problem? What have we agreed upon so far? Time is running out; can we pull some solid ideas together from our discussion?

• Evaluating the meeting at its close. Leadership and membership should know "how to make the best use of group sessions designed for genuine communication and joint decision" (ref. 16). They should ask themselves whether the particular meeting, in its planned format, was desirable, and whether it related to the auxiliary's problems, needs, and goals. "The objective of each meeting is to motivate human activities. Each individual who attends knows the topics and/or problems, and has given them the best thought of which he is capable. As a result of all the minds involved, the meeting concludes with a better solution than any one member had conceived at the outset" (ref. 17).

General Membership Meetings

Some general principles underlie the designing and conducting of effective membership meetings. Because they are multipurpose vehicles for problem solving, leadership training, membership education, and the stimulation of membership participation, it is imperative that the planning of such meetings receive priority consideration by both leadership and membership. The programming of meetings in relation to selection of subject matter and speakers, membership's role in program design, techniques of presentation, and the actual arrangement and conducting of the meeting are all influential factors in creating effective meetings, which, in turn, maintain membership interest and attendance.

The lack of attendance can be a cause for concern in many auxiliaries. Because a number of qualifying factors influence attendance figures, however, each auxiliary should analyze its individual situation to determine just how serious its attendance problem really is, or if it even exists. For example, when general membership meetings fail to produce at least 50 per cent attendance, on the average, it could be an appropriate time for the membership relations and membership education committees, and perhaps the entire membership body, to review programming and policies regarding membership participation in auxiliary affairs.

Although attendance of less than 50 per cent may be a danger signal, attendance of 50 per cent at membership meetings can be considered quite adequate — in certain circumstances. A qualifying factor could be the inactive members who swell the membership ranks by virtue of paying dues, but whose obligation to the auxiliary does not extend beyond this act. Included in this category are senior members of long-established auxiliaries who, after years of dedication, have ceased to participate actively in the group's affairs, or younger auxilians who wish to support the work of the auxiliary financially without contributing time and energy. Among members in the active category, some will attend meetings according to their preference for the subject matter.

"The auxiliary leadership should be concerned only with the lack of attendance of the active members. They are the ones who are the doers, the pace-setters, the problem-solvers, or the problem-makers. Thus in evaluating attendance at meetings, the formula should be: total membership minus all inactive categories . . . minus the occasional attenders and the emergency absentees (illness, and so forth), minus the inevitable one-time-only attenders. The result equals good attendance" (ref. 16).

An astute membership relations committee will have sufficient knowledge of the individuals constituting its particular group to develop realistic expectations concerning attendance at meetings. Attendance can never be compulsory; it must emanate voluntarily from a membership that has been motivated by stimulating, well-presented programs, encompassing both the business and the educational aspects of the auxiliary's affairs.

Programming

Successful meetings draw their strengths from thoughtful programming. When provocative, sometimes controversial subject matter, relevant to the purpose of the auxiliary, is presented dynamically, the result is greater attendance at meetings, more enthusiastic response from members, and increased participation in the work of the group. Even the business session of membership meetings can be designed to elicit interest, and it should receive particular attention in its development and presentation. Business matters requiring discussion and action by the group fulfill membership's expectations that it is attending meetings to participate.

The membership education committee bears a major responsibility for developing programs that will accomplish these goals. It is not alone in this responsibility, however. Building effective programs, and therefore meetings, should create a productive membership. For this reason, members should be actively involved in developing the types of programs most beneficial and appealing to them.

Brainstorming

Shared responsibility can be accomplished by periodic brainstorming meetings focusing on the creation of interesting and motivational programs and methods of presentation. All members could be invited to express their views on the subject, in addition to offering observations on leadership's techniques of handling membership and annual meetings and the actual educational value of present programming. A questionnaire, submitted to members a week or so prior to this special meeting and brought along with them, could stimulate thinking along appropriate channels.

Focusing group attention on this important area of auxiliary affairs can be a unifying experience for membership and leadership alike. Members should be made to feel that everyone's opinion counts and receives consideration, that everyone's input is valuable and necessary. This attitude on the part of leadership can help to eliminate the feeling that all decisions within the auxiliary are made by the board and that the general membership is expected to approve decisions "after the fact."

The technique of holding brainstorming meetings can be utilized in confronting other major problems such as recruitment, new uses for auxiliary funds, new functions for auxilians, expanding and improving the auxiliary's community relations program, and other subjects of concern. For further information on utilizing the technique of brainstorming, auxilians should consult books and magazine articles in local libraries.

Committee Members as Resources

Through their personal and professional contacts, individuals serving on the membership education committee are obvious resources for obtaining knowledgeable and dynamic speakers for membership meetings. Beginning with the institution and working outward to community, city, state, and national organizations, committee members should be able to assemble representative, informative speakers and to offer suggestions on stimulating subject matter. Other resources, close at hand, include the assorted committees of the auxiliary, which can provide ongoing assistance in programming, and the most recent past chairman of the membership education committee, who should be able to contribute attendance figures and reactions to the previous year's programs.

Variety

Variety in the format of programs is essential. The use of guest speakers can be supplemented with audiovisual elements, which are an excellent supportive technique for presenting information and for varying the method of presentation. Motion picture and slide films, tape recordings, videotapes, and flip charts can add new dimensions to the educational process and the effectiveness of programs.

Using various formats in programming is also a productive technique for increasing membership participation in meetings. The traditionally formal lecture, followed by a brief question-and-answer period, has been expanded in most contemporary organizations into the open forum, in which the mood is informal and the audience is encouraged to engage in direct dialog with the speaker following the presentation. An extension of this method is the symposium, which consists of brief talks by several speakers, followed by questions from the audience. A panel discussion, using auxiliary members as panelists who debate subjects with a guest speaker, or a panel of experts who engage in debate, followed by audience participation, would be similarly effective in sustaining membership interest.

A sample board meeting of the auxiliary, during which business is actually transacted, could be staged yearly as a demonstration to the general membership and as a device for including members in the inner workings of the auxiliary. Intra-auxiliary workshops on significant subjects, held periodically, provide further diversification in programming and offer in-depth educational experiences.

An efficiently functioning membership education committee should be able to announce the year's meeting dates and the majority of program subjects at the beginning of the auxiliary's year. (Speakers can be added later.) The arrangements should be flexible enough, however, to permit changes or additions when important subjects or events arise that deserve inclusion.

Techniques of Presentation

Given stimulating, relevant subject matter, an auxiliary's programs need forceful, concise presentation of material if membership is to be aroused and maintained. All participants in the program should have a prior and thorough understanding of what is expected of each of them, specifically. It is the responsibility of the membership education committee to communicate this information, well in advance, to guest speakers, auxiliary officers, committee chairmen, and members who will be making keynote presentations and reports or handling special arrangements. This careful preplanning can help to ensure a coordinated, smoothly functioning event, with participants oriented to their appropriate roles within the context of the meeting.

Whether the speakers are auxilians conducting the business session of membership meetings, members of the institution's professional staff offering orientation on new services or expanded programs, or guest lecturers providing educational information on a variety of topics, the principles of presentation remain the same:

• The speaker should focus precisely on the subject.
• The speaker should finish within a predetermined period of time.
• The presentation should be designed to be as interesting and provocative as possible.
• Members' response to the information offered, including further exploration of ideas and discussion of differences, should be encouraged.

- The presentation should begin with some provocative comment that gets the audience's attention and focuses it on the subject.
- Introductions of speakers should be brief and concise.
- Experienced speakers should be encouraged to make their presentations extemporaneous whenever possible.

Arranging and Conducting Meetings

Physical arrangements for meetings should be handled by the membership education committee, with attention to setting up the meeting room properly. This includes providing seating for the audience and appropriate equipment for the program following the business session (speaker's rostrum, table and chairs to accommodate a panel discussion, and so forth).

The type of meeting should determine the kind of seating for those attending. For example, a small number of persons — such as a discussion or workshop group from an institute or seminar — could be accommodated at a large, round table. This creates a feeling of intimacy and can heighten the interchange between participants. Lecture meetings would more appropriately use the regular audience-style seating arrangement.

All equipment, particularly audiovisual, should be checked in advance to ascertain whether it is in working order. If coffee or other refreshments are to be served during or after the meeting, the required equipment and food also should be assured ahead of time.

Various elements should be considered by the membership education committee when it makes arrangements for membership meetings.

Frequency and Time

The frequency of such meetings and the time of day they occur are important factors. They depend upon (1) the size of the geographic area served by the institution and the traveling time required to reach meetings, (2) the number of members currently involved in auxiliary committee work that requires conscientious attention and attendance at committee meetings, (3) other types and frequency of meetings held by the auxiliary, (4) other volunteer activities within the community that may demand the time and commitment of auxilians, (5) the members' expressed attitudes toward how often and when meetings are held, and (6) the current composition of the auxiliary in terms of the number of members having full-time jobs and the auxiliary's interest in encouraging new membership among working women and men.

Some auxiliaries opt for monthly meetings on the basis of past experience with attendance and interest; others consider bimonthly or trimonthly meetings to be more than sufficient. If an auxiliary has active committees that meet fairly frequently, the demands upon members may already be considerable. In addition to committee meetings, there may be the special membership meetings discussed earlier, intra-auxiliary workshops, and meetings with other local auxiliaries on a community or regional basis. For the auxiliary's officers, there are, of course, the board meetings.

The time of day or evening during which meetings are held relates directly to the convenience of the members and the availability of meeting space. Although many members may be satisfied with the established meeting time, others might appreciate a periodic change of hour to suit *their* convenience. Most auxiliaries meet in a room provided at the institution. It is advisable, however, to vary the meeting place and arrangements occasionally. For example, if most membership gatherings follow a straight meeting format, a stimulating variation could be a luncheon or dinner meeting, held in a private room of an appropriate restaurant. Flexibility in scheduling meeting time and location is an important asset for the auxiliary, in terms of serving the members' interest and providing variety.

Length

This sensitive subject, a problem for many auxiliaries, has no single or simple solution. Three hours filled with stimulating presentations and membership participation can seem too brief, whereas one hour of an unimaginative program can be the breaking point for the most tolerant members.

Because it is a relative matter, based upon the individual auxiliary's need and capability to inform, educate, and motivate action, it is appropriate here only to suggest that each auxiliary experiment until it establishes that "reasonable" amount of time for its own group. Once determined, however, the method of operation should be flexible enough to permit deviations from the norm.

This double standard, as it were, concerning the duration of meetings consists of two propositions. The first is that meetings must function within a prescribed time period: they should begin and end as scheduled. Unfortunately, this is where auxiliaries experience difficulty. Adhering to this principle requires discipline, which, in turn, is rooted in sound planning. An initial step toward this disciplined approach is for the membership education committee to announce the time limits for each meeting in advance, and then purposefully to fit the program into this framework. Further, the committee should create an awareness among program participants, whether guest speakers or auxilians, of the importance of adhering to their allotted time slots. The auxiliary president should assume responsibility for tactfully moving the program along, indicating to participants, when necessary, that it is time to summarize. This awareness of time is particularly important to auxilians who are conducting the business session of the meeting, because it is rude and annoying for guest speakers to be kept "waiting in the wings" while the affairs of the auxiliary grind on.

However, there *is* another side to this coin — that it is poor policy to restrict legitimate discussion by the membership about auxiliary matters, or to arbitrarily cut off a productive discussion between guest speaker and audience just because time is running out. This is the second proposition regarding duration of meetings: the auxiliary should be able to accommodate unexpected or spontaneous events within the framework of the meeting and to recognize when such events are sufficiently significant to justify an expansion of the original meeting time. Some other alternatives are to devote an entire meeting to business, to anticipate the need for lengthy discussion, or to postpone that discussion to the next meeting or even a special meeting. Each auxiliary must learn, through actual experience, what constitutes appropriate time allotments for the various elements in a meeting program. More important than whether a meeting ends on time is the necessity for it to end decisively.

The Business Session

Perhaps the most challenging aspect of conducting meetings

relates to the business session, that all-important vehicle for dealing with the internal management and external affairs of the auxiliary. Because the responsibility for the conducting and content of the business session rests with the president and board of directors, it is within their province to make it either a productive and educationally satisfying experience or an endurance test. When the business session is used to stimulate communication between leadership and membership, to gain acceptance of program, to initiate action, and to train potential leadership, it is serving its ultimate purpose.

Even with their confining elements, business sessions offer ample opportunity for the auxiliary president to establish the tone of such meetings at the beginning and for other leaders to reinforce it during the proceedings. The tone consists of a number of aspects: a positive attitude; a feeling of informality (but still consistent with use of parliamentary procedure) ; a sincere desire to involve members as active participants in the business of the auxiliary; an impersonal approach to discussing differences of opinion; the ability to utilize certain meeting management techniques, such as the question, to stimulate contributions from all the members; the establishment of the meeting's goals at the very start; and a clear concept of priorities regarding what must be accomplished during the meeting (as set out in the agenda). A carefully planned and well-thought-out agenda establishes the direction of the meeting and helps reinforce the efforts of the officers to set the tone of the meeting. For a detailed description of the development of agendas, see Chapter 10, "Records and Reports."

The Little Courtesies

It is a gracious gesture on the part of the auxiliary for a representative of the membership education committee to meet guest speakers upon their arrival at the airport or at their hotel and escort them to the meeting. Similarly, new auxiliary members attending a meeting for the first time should be contacted in advance by a representative of the membership relations committee and greeted by that person as they enter the room for their initial meeting. These courtesies, which establish more immediate rapport, help people to feel comfortable and accepted in new situations.

Annual Meetings

A special opportunity is afforded the auxiliary through the medium of the annual meeting. It has a potential for considerable impact on the membership and community, because within the span of several hours the annual meeting is capable of drawing together diverse individuals on behalf of a community institution, helping them to reaffirm their common purpose and providing interpretation of the institution's goals, current and future, to a representative portion of that community. An annual meeting is the wrap-up, the culminating event of a year's accomplishments and, simultaneously, the appropriate point from which to make projections for future achievements.

As stated in the model bylaws in Appendix A, the auxiliary is required to hold an annual meeting for the purpose of electing and installing officers, receiving the annual reports of officers, and conducting such other business as may properly come before the meeting. In addition to these organizational purposes, an annual meeting also can serve to bring the members closer together in a more thorough understanding of the auxiliary and its work, can have public relations value by providing an opportunity to publicize the auxiliary's various programs on behalf of the institution and the community and helping the auxiliary to win new friends who will support its work, and can provide a reason for conducting a social affair. An auxiliary's annual meeting is frequently a mixture of all these objectives.

The bylaws also recommend that the annual meeting be held about a month following the end of the auxiliary's fiscal year, which should coincide with the fiscal year of the institution. The annual meeting generally takes the place of the auxiliary's regular meeting for that month. Notice of the meeting should be given to the membership approximately 30 days in advance. The length of the annual meeting will depend, of course, upon the type of program being conducted.

Inviting community representatives, or even the general public, to attend the annual meeting is an excellent way to inform and involve the very people that the institution is serving. It is also a natural vehicle for recruiting new auxilians or individuals for the institution's department of volunteer services. To ensure this attendance, invitations should be sent to key individuals and organizations within the community, and a schedule of advance publicity worked out with the institution's public relations-community relations department, if there is one. Otherwise, the auxiliary's community relations committee should work with the institution's chief executive or other staff person who has previously established channels of communication with the media.

A subcommittee of the membership education committee can be appointed to handle the program and physical arrangements for this special event. It would be advisable for this committee to review other community organizational activities during the month of the projected annual meeting in order to avoid conflicting dates. The subcommittee should also approach the membership on the type of annual meeting desired, such as a banquet and meeting combination, with or without guest speaker; a straight meeting format, with or without guest speaker, followed by a social hour and refreshments; or an annual meeting held in tandem with a "Health Day" at the institution, offering educational seminars on subjects relevant to the community. Depending upon the final determination, arrangements should then be made, well in advance, to obtain appropriate meeting space, equipment, food service, and related necessities.

Business Program

The program for the business portion of the annual meeting should offer an in-depth view of the auxiliary's accomplishments and plans via reports of officers and committee chairmen. However, care should be taken not to overload the agenda.

A suggested sequence for this segment is as follows:
1. Annual report from the president.
2. Reports from the president-elect, vice presidents for service and community relations, secretary, treasurer, and various committee chairmen.
3. Election and installation of new officers.
4. Recogniton of retiring officers and committee chairmen.

President's Report

The president's annual report should be a concise and interesting presentation of the auxiliary's achievements during the past year and immediate objectives for the year ahead, condensed from the more detailed, printed version of the auxiliary's annual report, which is distributed to the membership, the institution, and the community. If desired, it can be extended to include the auxiliary's long-range plans for the next five to ten years, to provide a more comprehensive outlook. Time limit for this report should not exceed 15 to 20 minutes, if possible. The president's presentation can be supplemented with visuals if they will contribute clarity and interest. As the presiding officer for the annual meeting, the president is responsible for keeping the proceedings moving in a well-paced manner.

Other Reports

A succession of official reports can be anathema to an annual meeting. To avoid this possibility, the reports of other officers and committee chairmen should be duplicated and distributed to the membership prior to the meeting, requiring only that the reports be accepted at the meeting itself. During the meeting, officers and committee chairmen should be presented personally and granted the privilege of requesting action on their respective reports. Although this portion of the program should be brief, time should be allotted for possible discussion.

When these reports are prepared for advance distribution, they should be arranged according to the structural relationships that exist between officers and committee chairmen. For example, the president-elect coordinates committees concerned with the auxiliary's internal functions; therefore, her report would be tied into the work of such committees as those on finance, membership education, and membership relations. Similarly, the vice presidents for service and community relations are concerned with the auxiliary's external affairs, so their reports would focus on the committees for community relations, volunteer services, legislation, gift and coffee shop, and so forth. By structuring these reports in their appropriate relationships to the internal and external affairs of the auxiliary, better understanding is promoted among members of the ways in which the auxiliary operates.

Election and Installation of New Officers

These two functions, which are provided for in the bylaws, are necessary elements in an annual meeting. The traditional activity of installing officers, which occurs after the election at the auxiliary's annual meeting, provides the opportunity for the auxiliary to accomplish several important purposes. In addition to officially marking the change in administration, the installation also permits the outgoing president to express appreciation to fellow officers, committee chairmen, and the membership; allows the officers to acknowledge the membership's contribution, and for membership to return the compliment; and helps to motivate new officers and the membership toward greater achievement in the year ahead.

Conducting an actual installation ceremony is a matter that each auxiliary must determine individually. It is not a legal necessity, because the results of the auxiliary's elections automatically cancel the former administration and its authority — unless the auxiliary's bylaws indicate otherwise.

If the auxiliary wishes to have a brief, simple procedure, in which the gavel is handed over to the new president, and the incoming and outgoing officers are invited to say a few words, this may well suffice. For those auxiliaries that still prefer the more traditional and elaborate type of proceeding, this, too, is appropriate if it satisfies a need for ceremony that the membership recognizes and wishes to perpetuate. However, with the abundance of material that is usually covered in the annual meeting, it would be wise, perhaps, to reconsider the length and complexity of the ceremony in terms of the members' patience and retention of interest.

Recognition of Service

Formal recognition of retiring officers and committee chairmen gives psychological gratification to those who have contributed to the work of the auxiliary and permits the membership to express appreciation. Recognition of individual contributions of members should be limited to brief acknowledgments. This is particularly applicable to committee chairmen, who may be tempted to use their annual reports as a vehicle for thanking each committee member individually and profusely. A more efficient way of handling this situation is for the chairman to thank her committee as a group, *during* the meeting, and permit the written version of her report, which is sent out in advance to the membership, to contain individual acknowledgments.

Special Program

Official Presentation

The business portion of the annual meeting can be followed

by a presentation by the institution's chief executive or by the chairman or president of the board of trustees. This is an excellent opportunity for a representative of the institution to provide a comprehensive view of the institution-auxiliary relationship and to describe its continuing existence in terms of present and future needs.

Feature Presentation

The auxiliary may determine that a portion of the program should be devoted to highlighting the institution for some special reason (expansion or initiation of services with corresponding impact on the hospital, auxiliary, and community), or to presenting a priority topic of information that will be highly influential in directing the activities of the institution and the auxiliary for the coming year (for example, new health care legislation). Such feature presentations should be carefully planned. Appropriate speakers should be contacted sufficiently early to enable them to prepare incisive and insightful lectures. Speakers can be drawn from the institution's administrative or medical staff, from local health organizations or educational institutions, or from state or national organizations.

Recruitment Meetings

Periodically, auxiliary membership meetings should include guests from throughout the community, in order to recruit new auxilians and individuals for the institution's department of volunteer services and to provide a basic educational orientation on the work of the auxiliary and the institution. Invitations can be extended to members of the institution's staff and individuals serving in the department of volunteer services, other auxiliaries in the area, volunteers and staff from other community organizations, and friends and neighbors. An effort should be made to include men, senior citizens, and young persons in these open meetings to provide diversification in the potential volunteer force serving the institution.

Community Meetings

There may be occasions when the auxiliary will want or need to appeal to the community at large. Such a situation is described in Chapter 12, "How to Start an Auxiliary," in which a mass meeting is called to present the auxiliary's organizational plans to the public and to recruit members. Or the auxiliary may determine, in conjunction with the institution, that community action is urgently needed to effect changes in current health care legislation. The auxiliary, therefore, invites the community to a public meeting to provide education on the issues, to relate these issues to the community's health care needs, and to stimulate support in the appropriate direction.

When meetings of this type are initiated, the auxiliary will want to work in close cooperation with the institution's administrative staff and public relations-community relations department in order to organize and promote them.

chapter 10
Records and Reports

Good records are the key to sound management.

Mrs. Harry Milton,
former chairman,
Council on Hospital Auxiliaries
(now Committee on Volunteers),
American Hospital Association

Organization records are the basis for
club activities and action.
They constitute the history of the group.

John B. Shepperd, in
The President's Guide to Club and
Organization Management and Meetings,
New York: Hawthorn Books, Inc., 1961

An auxiliary's history is written in its records and reports. This ongoing narrative is maintained by those persons who are charged with the responsibility for recording and reporting all relevant decisions and activities. Because these auxilians rotate in and out of their elected and appointed offices, it is necessary that a clearly defined and consistent approach to record taking and to maintenance and techniques of reporting be sustained. This approach should facilitate personnel change, making the assumption of new jobs simpler, provide for continuity in the furnishing of relevant information to each successive leadership group, and transmit the specific kind of information needed by leadership to maintain an effectively functioning auxiliary.

All the auxiliary's activities and decisions depend, to some extent, on what has gone before. To utilize past experience to the fullest in making decisions for the present and future, it is essential that the recording and reporting of the auxiliary's affairs be accurate, complete, and perceptively handled. This implies more than a pedestrian approach to recording and reporting; it demands, in effect, that these processes be creative, capable of stimulating a positive response from membership, and thereby acting as an impetus to action.

Effective recording and reporting are important factors in the sound management of the auxiliary. If reports are action-oriented, offering a pithy extraction of the most significant elements from well-developed records, they will serve their appropriate educational purpose. The retention of records and reports — discussed in detail at the end of this chapter — and their provision to successive leadership are equally important aspects. By making such information accessible and encouraging its use by leadership, certain techniques are established for both the approach to record taking and the utilization of the information contained therein for development into reports.

For purposes of clarification, it should be noted that recording and reporting are interrelated processes: one without the other is functionless. The recording process secures the information that provides the basis for the report. Recording should be a highly selective process, however, to help ensure the report's relevance. Once the report has been written, by use of further selectivity and focusing techniques, it requires an audience, whether readers or listeners, to give it life. The activity of reporting to *someone* places the report in the category of a communications tool.

It is important to differentiate among those who record and maintain information, those who use this information in the presentation of reports, either verbal or written, and those to whom such reports are given. Within the auxiliary's structure, the secretary, the treasurer, and the committee secretaries are the recorders and keepers of the auxiliary's history. Responsibility for the reporting process is assumed by the auxiliary's president, who reports to the board of directors and the membership, in addition to the institution's chief executive and governing board; vice presidents and committee chairmen, who report to the board of directors and the membership when appropriate; and the auxiliary's secretary and treasurer, whose periodic reports are channeled to the board of directors and membership. How well these individuals fulfill the responsibilities of recording and reporting depends upon how thoroughly and skillfully they have been oriented to the techniques that produce truly informative communications.

The records and reports of primary importance to an auxiliary are:

1. Minutes for its own board, committee, and membership meetings (minutes are classified as records).
2. Officers' reports.
3. Annual reports, incorporating the annual audited statement on financial status from the auxiliary's treasurer (annual financial and budgetary statements are classified as records).
4. Periodic reports to the community on the auxiliary's progress in specific programs and projects, and use of contributed funds. For more frequent communication, the auxiliary's newsletter can be utilized.

The records and reports of secondary importance include various types of information that serve as tools in the development of the primary records and reports. Agendas for meetings, interim financial reports, committee progress reports, and the personal notebooks maintained by the auxiliary's president and committee chairmen — these interim records and reports all play a supportive role in the preparation of a profile of the auxiliary's yearly activities.

All these recording and reporting activities, if functioning optimally, can provide the continuity that links each year's leadership group with the next, contribute to better integrated communications within the auxiliary, and facilitate the auxiliary's communications with institution and community.

Minutes

Minutes are the ongoing narrative of the auxiliary — the record of decisions made and progress achieved, the vehicle for continuity. Depending upon the approach to their recording and utilization, minutes can be a truly effective tool for communicating the essential facts about the auxiliary's operations. As the records of current and past activities, minutes "are indispensable to sound business management, planning and follow-up. Accurate minutes portray the thinking of the group and the contributions of individual members" (ref. 40).

The purpose of taking minutes is to summarize meeting activities in such a manner that the minutes serve as informative documents, capable of creating and sustaining interest in the auxiliary's operations from meeting to meeting. Highly definitive, action-oriented minutes can also help an auxiliary to achieve the particular objectives of the succeeding meeting.

For the purpose of conciseness, and because the recording of minutes is a similar process — whether it be during board, membership, or committee meetings — techniques for recording that apply to all these situations are presented here.

Listening to, interpreting, and recording information effectively are skills that usually must be acquired, especially as they apply to the often rapid conversational give-and-take that characterizes meetings.

Selectivity and concentration are key words in the recording of minutes. The total process is further enhanced by an almost intuitive recognition of what is pertinent and what is not. This approach to recording surpasses mere note-taking on what transpired during a meeting. It concentrates on the content of the meeting rather than the procedures. The minutes should reflect what the meeting produces and recommends — decisions made, decisions not made, progressive or status quo situations. "The recording secretary should understand that voluminous word-for-word playbacks or boiled-down abstractions are not desirable. Good minutes reflect the meeting's highlights" (ref. 54).

In recording the gist of the discussion, the essential points, the secretary need not list details unless they are really relevant, but must learn to "completely concentrate on the thread of the discussion." Eventually, "intent listening will help the vital points to come to the surface and identify themselves" (ref. 55).

Thomas A. Piraino, vice president for commercial development, Gregory Industries, states: "The individual who records meetings and issues minutes should think of himself as participating in an active executive activity, rather than passively recording an event. The difference is a key to the effectiveness of the records for stimulating action" (ref. 45).

The basic procedural content of minutes should include the date of the meeting, the location, the time of the meeting's beginning and adjournment, a statement that the meeting was duly called on proper notice, a list of those attending, and the names of the chairman and the recording secretary.

In addition, the minutes should cover the motions carried; the number of members voting affirmatively, negatively, or abstaining; the resolutions adopted; summaries of any substantive discussion, even if no decision was reached; specific assignments to individuals or committees, with provisions for reporting progress by certain dates; and summations of reports presented by officers and committee chairmen. Each item of business on the agenda should be considered and numbered separately in the minutes.

Prior to the meeting, the secretary should become familiar with the objectives to be accomplished, reports to be presented, and so forth. "This premeeting orientation will make it possible to outline in one's mind the probable important aspects of the meeting, and give a sense of direction to note-taking in anticipation of writing minutes. . . . The degree to which meetings accomplish objectives depends upon many things outside of the control of the minute-taker. If the minute-taker has done his homework, however, he can spot, in the discussions, those conclusions and recommendations which most closely relate to the meeting's objectives. In the minutes, these should be clearly and concisely presented so that the attention of readers is focused on such items" (ref. 45). Regardless of the length of time spent in discussion during a meeting, the degree of importance determines the amount of attention items receive in the minutes.

Key conclusions, recommendations, and assignments should not be obscured by background information or a storytelling style, both of which make it difficult to develop required action among the membership, according to Piraino (ref. 45). A special section can be set aside within the minutes of every meeting for noting assignments, along with the names of persons responsible and the deadlines for performance.

An effective technique for ensuring accurate interpretation of and emphasis on pertinent conclusions reached during a meeting is for the recording secretary to orally summarize a particular point that may have been unclearly defined during discussion. This technique causes meeting participants to concur, on the spot, about the correct interpretation. This practice should be used sparingly, and only when the subject matter has been sufficiently developed to merit oral summarization. By requesting interpretation of specific points that seem highly relevant to the current discussion, the recording secretary also helps the group to determine whether that point is valuable enough to include in the minutes.

This same predilection for accuracy should be reflected in the recorder's ability to duplicate, in writing, each motion that has been made, seconded, and carried, or each resolution that has been adopted — exactly as it has been stated. If necessary, the recording secretary should call for a halt to any vote or proceeding until it can be entered, word for word, in her notes.

The conclusions or recommendations of formal written or oral reports should be summarized in the minutes. A brief statement on the discussion or activities that led to such recommendations or conclusions can be included if it is truly pertinent to achieving an understanding of the situation. "Putting the action-oriented parts of formal reports into minutes forces consideration of such items, and leads to action" (ref. 45).

The preparation of minutes is facilitated by the use of the agenda, for it provides the basic direction that the recorder will be following. When the writing of the minutes has been completed, the recorder submits them to the appropriate meeting chairman for approval as to substance and accuracy. Minutes should be distributed to the general membership or to board or committee members as soon as possible following the meeting, while the material is still fresh and easily recalled. Copies of the minutes of auxiliary membership and board meetings should be provided to the institution's governing board and chief executive. These minutes, in addition to minutes of committee meetings, should also be retained in the auxiliary's official files.

Prior to auxiliary meetings, members should be encouraged to review the minutes from the previous meeting, as well as the agenda for the upcoming meeting, in order to orient themselves to the exact point of progress reached by the auxiliary in regard to its various functions. The reading aloud of previous meeting minutes during a current meeting is a formality that generally is waived. It is assumed that auxilians — whether board or committee members or general membership — will be responsible for examining these minutes prior to the meeting and need only vote their approval or disapproval. The exception to this procedure occurs when corrections of the minutes are offered. If such corrections are interpretive in nature, there should be a discussion on the suggested changes prior to substitution. When corrections are accepted, the secretary must note them for inclusion in the minutes of the present meeting. Then the minutes of the previous meeting can be approved as corrected.

The recording secretary's responsibility should not be limited to her "ability to distinguish between relevant and irrelevant discussions, and skill in developing records that portray an accurate picture of the work of the [group]." Essential as these qualities are, they "should not preclude her participation in the committee's or group's deliberations." She may have a "special contribution to make by her careful analysis of previous discussion and actions of the committee" (ref. 19).

Minutes can play a significant role in stimulating an action-oriented response: "Without minimizing the importance of pre-meeting preparation or meeting leadership and participation, my thesis is that coordinated group action resulting from meetings can be dramatically improved through more effective postmeeting action, and that the key to such action is better writing and better administrative handling of minutes" (ref. 45).

Reports: Principles and Techniques

The primary purposes of reporting are to communicate relevant information to the auxiliary's membership and institution in the most effective manner possible and to accomplish the desired goal of this process, which is motivation of membership to take certain courses of action. Good reporting techniques, involving both preparation and presentation, can provide the impetus that puts this process in gear and, with the assistance of leadership, can keep it functioning productively.

Whether written or oral, good reports avoid such characteristics as sloppiness in preparation and presentation, provision of information that is neither conclusive nor informative, and unnecessary repetition of facts. Prolonged rather than concise presentation of reports and the use of reporting as a form of personal ego gratification also serve to diminish their ultimate effectiveness.

Good reports are also accurate ones. The value of a report is reduced in direct proportion to the number of errors contained within it. There is little rationale for presenting a report if the accuracy of the information has not been verified. Correct identification of persons, committees, institutional departments, community organizations, and dates, as well as proper interpretation of the proceedings, are all essential elements in preparing a report and ensuring its validity.

Certain principles apply to the preparation and presentation of all reports. A major technique to increase the effectiveness of reporting is to use highlights of activities rather than extremely detailed narration. Although it is important to provide a rationale for the conclusions and recommendations within a report — outlining opposing viewpoints and alternative suggestions — it is equally important to learn how to summarize, to include only significant points, and to be concise. This approach is similar to that used in the preparation of minutes.

The need for brief, comprehensible, and nonrepetitive reporting becomes particularly apparent during meetings in which a series of reports is presented orally. If the report includes little variety, lengthy oratory, or nonessential information, it will merge colorlessly into the next report, leaving the audience uninterested. Consequently, the audience's opportunity for education is diminished. Reports should inform; they should not have to be endured. Unless the primary purposes of reports are served, there is no real reason to present them.

The frequency and rationale for reporting are determined by a few simple standards: something important and timely is being imparted, board or membership approval is required in order to proceed with a project, or a significant stage of progress in a program or project has been reached. The assumption that officers or committee chairmen are obligated, by tradition, to present reports at *every* board, membership, or committee meeting is unrealistic and impractical.

Reports of Officers and Committee Chairmen

Officers and committee chairmen are responsible for reporting to the auxiliary's board and membership. The president also reports to the institution's chief executive and governing board. As communicators of the auxiliary's essential information, officers share the obligation to use effective reporting techniques and to concern themselves with such questions as: How can reports be developed to most successfully communicate the information that the auxiliary and the institution need to know? How often should reports be given? What are the justifications for giving reports? Should the presentation be written or oral?

Reports to the Board of Directors

Reporting to the auxiliary's board is, basically, a request for a decision or information on the subject matter being presented. The type of subject matter that qualifies for board attention should involve such major areas of concern as the initiation of a comprehensive program or project, questions on policy matters, the need for additional funds from the auxiliary to operate programs, or the official response of the institution's chief executive or governing board to an auxiliary proposal. All these matters require board discussion, exchange of information, action, or approval.

In essence, however, those reporting are *sharing* their concerns with other board members, rather than making formal reports. They are also sharing information on the current status of auxiliary projects, keeping the board up to date. Their aim is to draw upon the experience and expertise of board members, to use them as a sounding board for problems, and to obtain the kind of feedback that will enable the respective officers and committee chairmen to proceed with their work.

Matters brought before the board for discussion should, when necessary for clarity, be supplemented with a written report supplied to board members in advance of meetings. Proposals for new ventures, particularly, should be written up in detail and distributed for prior examination. This procedure facilitates decision making. If the proposal is accepted by the board, the written report can then be used as the basis for developing a presentation for the membership or the institution at a later date.

Reports to Membership

Reports by officers or committee chairmen at membership meetings should be concerned with policies and programs that have reached a conclusion — either successful or unsuccessful — or have reached a decisive stage in their development. The peaks and valleys are of interest, whereas the plateaus usually are not. The term *progress*, within this context, should be defined as actually offering new developments since the last report was presented; otherwise there is no purpose for its inclusion. (The subject of progress reports by committee chairmen to the auxiliary's board and membership is described in detail later in this chapter, in the section entitled "Tools." Committee progress reports are an interim type of information used in the development of the primary records and reports discussed here.) In some instances, it may be advisable and timesaving for written reports to be submitted to membership in advance of meetings.

Other qualifications that make such reporting appropriate are that the report is of special significance to the membership in terms of educational value or that the substance of the report requires group discussion and action. If the auxiliary president, the membership education committee, and committee chairmen work closely on establishing standards for the inclusion of reports in meeting programs, such reports will assume a more meaningful status when they *are* presented.

Responsibility for reporting to the general membership on recommendations and actions by the auxiliary's board of directors or the institution's governing board, and for gaining assent on major new programs, rests with the auxiliary's president, who is the communication link between the two entities. The president should also inform the membership about important proposals submitted to the auxiliary's board by committees, whether the board has approved such proposals or not. This action can stimulate a response from membership, thereby giving the board feedback on membership reaction. The president may also call upon committee chairmen to provide supportive data for the membership's consideration.

Financial Reports

Two major areas of accountability for the auxiliary's financial affairs are assumed by the auxiliary's treasurer: (1) the audited financial statements (income and expense and balance sheet) that are included in the auxiliary's annual report to its institution and community and (2) the interim financial reports to the auxiliary's board of directors. (The latter are discussed in the section entitled "Tools.")

In order for the annual financial statements to accurately and significantly reflect the current status of the auxiliary's finances, its financial commitments to the institution, and its success or failure in achieving its stated financial goals for the year, certain selected information should be gathered by the treasurer for inclusion. The financial statements, which represent a major aspect of the auxiliary's annual report, should focus upon the primary sources of revenue for the auxiliary, amount and categories of expenditure, comparison of revenue and expenditures, and current asset value of the auxiliary. If a deficit exists, the report should explain how it will be met. The statements should then compare this collection of data with budgeted estimates projected for the year, to facilitate appraisal of budgeting techniques. If desired, the previous year's figures can be compared to the current ones, category by category, to indicate any changes in financial situation.

All figures in the statements should be certified by an auditor, and the fact of this certification should be noted at the completion of the statements. It is preferable for an independent auditor to be used, if the auxiliary can afford these services. For a small auxiliary or one with a limited budget, the institution's auditor would be the logical choice.

Annual Reports

"An annual report may be an obligation, but it should also be regarded as an opportunity" (ref. 32).

As the traditional form of summary concerning the auxiliary's activities, the annual report has frequently played a narrowly defined role in communications, reaching only the institution's administrative staff and governing board and the auxiliary's membership. Supplied as "privileged information" to these inner audiences, the auxiliary's annual report often was not regarded as material for public consumption. The same situation existed concerning the annual reports of health care institutions in general, which, many times, received little, if any, circulation outside of the immediate hospital family.

The concept of responsibility to a public that is supplying financial and moral support for the work of health care institutions, however, has become a dominant theme, characterizing the relationships of these institutions and auxiliaries to their communities. This attitude is, to some extent, a response to the demands of an increasingly sophisticated public for exact knowledge of the ways in which contributed funds are spent and what such expenditures accomplish. The other motivating factor is that institutions and their auxiliaries realize that without public support they cannot function effectively and that in order to merit this support they must be willing to disclose their financial and operational affairs.

The auxiliary's annual report is a symbol of this accountability. Therefore, it should be utilized to the fullest as a primary opportunity to enhance communications among the auxiliary, the institution, and the community, and to serve many purposes for the auxiliary and the institution.

One of the most discerning and contemporary interpretations of this multipurpose function of the annual report has been expressed by Koestler: "When thoughtfully conceived, written, and produced to present a vivid portrait of your agency in action, it can simultaneously record the past, interpret the present, and provide an intriguing glimpse into the future. It can reinforce the loyalty of your existing constituency and attract new adherents and supporters. It can clarify and shape public attitudes on significant social problems and issues. It can identify changing trends, analyze and portray their impact on individuals, on groups, or on the community as a whole. And — in doing any or all of these things — it can reinforce your agency's image as an alert, useful, and constructive force for human betterment" (ref. 32).

An auxiliary's annual report is, in effect, a public relations vehicle capable of year-round impact, depending upon its use. It is an interpretative tool for telling the auxiliary's story to a wide assortment of publics. When incorporated into the institution's annual report, it can more strongly reinforce the link between auxiliary and institution in the public's mind.

It is strongly recommended that the auxiliary follow the procedure of integrating its annual report with its institution's rather than producing it as a separate entity. This viewpoint is expressive of the auxiliary's role as an integral part of its institution, both legally and philosophically. Because the auxiliary is a member of the institutional family, existing only to serve the institution, it is most appropriate that the summation of the auxiliary's yearly efforts be recorded within the context of the institution's annual report.

Audience

The potential audience for the annual report will influence the content, style, and format of the report itself. Therefore, distribution should be determined prior to the actual writing. Responsibility for developing the distribution list generally rests with the institution's public relations-community relations department, with input from the administrative staff, governing board, and auxiliary.

From the auxiliary's point of view, the core audience for the annual report is the auxiliary's membership, the institution's administration staff, governing board, medical staff, and employees. Their inclusion in the distribution helps to strengthen the relationship between the auxiliary and the institution's employees, by heightening their awareness of the connection between auxiliary and institution.

Because of its presumably close relationship with the community, the auxiliary should be in a position to suggest some significant groups and individuals as targets for the annual report outlets that the institution may not have considered. For example, the auxiliary might suggest that the annual report be channeled to agencies with which the auxiliary and the institution maintain cooperative relationships. Legislators and community leaders who may be influential in matters pertaining to health care could receive copies. The local media could be supplied with copies. The report might be sent to persons and organizations that provide annual support and to potential contributors, such as businesses, philanthropic foundations, and civic, educational, professional, fraternal, and other organizations.

Writing

For purposes of consistency, flow, and general maintenance of sanity, one person within the auxiliary — and one person only — should assume responsibility for the actual writing of the auxiliary's annual report. This approach avoids a final product that reads like a verbal patchwork quilt. Although it is often traditional for the auxiliary's president to be the author of the annual report, the material can be written by anyone in the auxiliary who possesses the writing ability.

Preparation for the actual writing process, however, should include the participation of a small group of auxilians who have convened specifically for the purpose of offering a broad spectrum of ideas on theme, content, approach, the use of visuals to illustrate the text, and related matters. This group may be a special one drawn together for this reason, or it may be the auxiliary's community relations committee that supplies the idea bank for the writer's efforts. Casual suggestions made at random by board members and auxilians throughout the year should also be considered during the final review of ideas, prior to writing.

Assuming that the auxiliary's annual report will be incorporated into the institution's, a general agreement should be reached with the institution's chief executive and public relations-community relations department concerning the auxiliary's concept of the report, suggested content, and space allotment for text and illustrations. When the writing has been completed, the annual report should be submitted by the auxiliary to its own officers and to the institution for final clearance on facts, figures, and interpretation.

Concerning style and tone in the creation of an annual report, "Warmth, simplicity, and directness make for the shortest road between you and your reader" (ref. 32). Annual reports create impact when they communicate these qualities to the reader with a sense of immediacy. Striving for comprehension is another aspect of writing that relates to style. "Specialists in readability research have developed scientific formulas dealing with sentence length, number of syllables per word, and related factors. For all practical purposes, their findings add up to this: short words, short sentences, and short paragraphs improve reader comprehension" (ref. 32).

Organization and Content

"The basic function of an annual report is to render an account of a single year's activities and expenditures" (ref. 32). This deceptively simple definition, realistically interpreted, implies a comprehensive roundup of all the auxiliary's work and accomplishments, reviewed with selective and fearless editorial ability. Such selectivity helps to ensure that the annual report contains sufficient information without being too all-inclusive, or a catchall for unnecessary data.

It is quite permissible and instructive to readers for the annual report to briefly mention the auxiliary's overall purposes and goals and relationship to the institution. Priority, however, demands that the annual report be concerned primarily with the actual accomplishments (and even failures) of the past 12 months; a determination of what really happened; and the significance of these events to the auxiliary, the institution, and the community. In distilling the essence from the year's activities, certain questions will arise, such as: Was the year characterized by rapidly evolving change, or was progress slow and steady, moving toward predetermined objectives? Were there major crises? Did the auxiliary achieve any of the principal goals it had established for itself?

It is essential to identify the dominant characteristics of the year that has passed and to ascertain progress toward future goals, in order to develop an overall theme for the annual report. The report serves, in effect, as a bridge between past and future, and the theme must make this connection real and vivid. "Organizational work is continuous, cumulative; whatever new directions are explored are the gradual outgrowth of experience and planning" (ref. 32). If the annual report is viewed as an effort to express this continuity, the result should be a powerful piece of communication.

The organizational outline for the contents of the annual report can be roughly represented as follows:

- Profile of the auxiliary, concisely stated, including fundamental goals and purposes, sources of its membership, identification of its board of directors and officers, geographic area served on behalf of its institution, and relationship to its institution, both organizationally and legally.
- Time period covered by the report, stated in terms of the auxiliary's fiscal year.
- Specific services rendered to institution and community, including statistics on number of individuals served and possible results of services. These services should be related to broader program goals, rather than being viewed as independent or unrelated projects.

- Roles auxilians played within the context of program activities to provide these services; also, their influence in the auxiliary's program planning.
- Financial statements (this subject is covered in the section entitled "Preparing Financial Reports").
- Analysis of the auxiliary's accomplishments during the past year. Did they fulfill expectations or fall short? If there were achievements *or* failures, what were the influential factors? In the event that financial or human resources weren't sufficient to carry the program through, how does the auxiliary plan to resolve the problem? Such candor helps to build credibility for the auxiliary's work in the public's mind. "A community-supported organization has the clear obligation to record its unresolved problems and its failures side by side with its triumphs. . . . The admission that a particular project failed to meet expectations convinces the reader that the agency has high standards, and makes him all the readier to believe whatever affirmative statements it may make about other areas of its work" (ref. 32).
- Identification of any significant national, regional, or local developments or major trends in health care delivery that have affected or will possibly affect the work of the auxiliary. Will changes in service to the institution and the community be necessary in coping with newly emerging needs in health care?
- Acknowledgment and description of the auxiliary's cooperative efforts with other community groups.
- Expression of appreciation, in general, for past financial and moral support by the community.

The Reader

A primary purpose of the annual report is to elicit response from the reader. The desired response may be membership in the auxiliary, financial contributions, service to the institution as a member of the department of volunteer services, activism through the promotion of health care legislation beneficial to the institution, or increased interest and moral support for the work of the auxiliary and the institution. If any of these responses are to be stimulated, the reader must be able to identify with the concerns and accomplishments presented to him.

Further, he must be given a specific, well-defined role to play in helping to advance the goals of the auxiliary and the institution. If he cannot see himself reflected in the report as a potential consumer of health care, and a member of the community that supports the institution, he will not become involved in the report's message, and therefore he will not be a potential resource for the institution in the areas mentioned.

The reader's knowledge of the auxiliary and the institution should never be taken for granted. The writer must put herself in the position of a person seeing this annual report from this particular organization for the first time, realizing that the reader could be someone who has intimate knowledge of the subject or, at the opposite end of the spectrum, someone who is totally uninformed. The opportunity for education offered by the annual report should be thoroughly exploited to cover these two extremes and all the levels of knowledge in between.

The Annual Report as a Separate Publication

For the auxiliary that is independently producing its own annual report, to be published separately from that of its institution, numerous determinations relating to the actual production aspects must be made. Whether an annual report is a simple, mimeographed document of a few pages, or a many paged, elaborate, multicolored presentation, replete with photos, drawings, and glossy paper, depends upon two factors: the budget and the hospital community. The individual means of expression for each auxiliary's annual report directly relates to the money available for the project and the probable or estimated response of the community served by the auxiliary and the institution.

If an institution is delivering health care primarily to a low-income community, an elaborate annual report would seem inappropriate, whether the auxiliary had the funds or not. Community residents might feel that the money would be better spent on additional, much needed health care services. Conversely if the auxiliary has a large budget allocation for such reports and is serving an affluent community, the auxiliary might believe that an impressive annual report would be exactly the correct way to thank contributors and keep them informed about the group's accomplishments and progress. Still another auxiliary may have the funds, but in principle feel that annual reports do not merit a large investment.

Other determinations the auxiliary must make in regard to production include determining the size of the printing or duplicating job; designing the report, which involves artwork and layout; choosing a printer or deciding where the duplicating should be done; and deciding on titles, illustrations, colors, type, and paper.

For the auxiliary that wishes to spend a minimal amount of money, the institution's duplicating resources should be utilized if possible. Whatever the process used, the auxiliary should take advantage of its institution's duplicating facility for the valuable assistance it can provide. Not only are costs reduced in the actual reproduction process, but also the staff involved in such work can offer suggestions on layout, design, and related matters.

When an auxiliary can afford to have its annual report printed by an outside firm, it will want to submit the job for bids from various printers in order to obtain the most reasonable price. A professional design firm might also be enlisted to provide consultation or to actually execute the artwork and layout for the report. It is possible that a design firm or the art department of a local advertising agency might contribute design services for a reduced fee, or for no charge, when a not-for-profit organization is seeking assistance.

To produce an annual report that is both professional in appearance and accurate in content, the auxiliary needs to adhere to a time schedule, working backward from the projected date of its annual meeting. Although there is no hard and fast rule about the time required to produce an annual report, a generous time allotment would be approximately four months, which would permit the following steps in the production process: (1) determine the overall theme, content, and design of the report; (2) write the report; (3) submit the completed draft to appropriate auxilians and representatives from the institution for review and clearance; (4) select illustrations and/or photographs and determine design and layout with artist and printer; (5) complete final rewriting, editing, and polishing of copy; and (6) submit final copy, art, and layout to printer. "The period of time required to produce an annual report depends on the length, sim-

plicity or complexity of the report. The only places not to skimp
. . . are in the planning and writing stages" (ref. 32).

The annual report should be released slightly in advance of the
auxiliary's annual meeting, to permit the membership to read it
ahead of time. It is suggested that for general distribution, however, the auxiliary's annual report be mailed out along with the
institution's. In this case, the institution will probably assume
responsibility for addressing the mailing labels or envelopes and
producing any special covering letters that may accompany the
joint mailing.

Promotion

If the auxiliary's annual report possesses any news of
significance, it should be brought to the attention of the local
media, accompanied by an explanatory press release. This promotion should be developed in cooperation with the institution's
department of public relations-community relations. In the event
that such assistance is not available from the institution, the
auxiliary should assume responsibility, through its community
relations committee and with the approval of administration, for
promoting its own annual report.

Some areas of information that may stimulate media interest
are (1) statistics showing significant trends in the community
services provided by auxilians; (2) results of innovative pilot
programs made possible, in part, by the auxiliary; (3) a new
approach to the solution of a difficult health care problem, in
which the auxiliary has played a significant role; (4) a change
in the institution's policy that will affect the auxiliary's functions
and have a decided impact on the community in terms of health
care provision; and (5) programs or projects sponsored by the
auxiliary that have real human interest value and demonstrate the
auxiliary's dedication to working directly with the community.

Alternative Approaches

Although the annual report is a tenacious tradition with
many auxiliaries, consideration should be given to some alternative approaches to this method of communication. Perhaps quarterly or semiannual reports, geared to the same audience as the
annual report, would be more effective in terms of timing and
frequency of exposure to the public. Included in this category

could be periodic reports to the community on the auxiliary's accomplishments in specific programs and projects and use of contributed funds. These various types of reports can all be distributed independently by the auxiliary or handled by the institution as special mailings.

Another possibility would be the use of audiovisual media for the transmission of such reports. Interesting departures from the usual printed format include a slide film, with narration provided by auxilians from a prepared script; a slide film with the sound track incorporated; or a tape cassette, providing sound only. Slide films can also serve as year-round promotional vehicles for the auxiliary's public education and fund-raising efforts, and can be accompanied by brief, supplementary written materials for distribution to the audiences.

Tools

Certain types of information qualify as tools in the development of primary records and reports. They serve interim purposes, providing the foundation for preparing minutes for meetings and summaries of the auxiliary's yearly activities, in addition to keeping the auxiliary's board and membership apprised of the current status of the organization's finances, projects, and programs. Within this category are agendas, interim financial reports, committee progress reports, and the personal notebooks that the auxiliary's president and committee chairmen maintain throughout their terms of office.

Agendas

"The importance of having an agenda prepared in advance cannot be overemphasized." An agenda is a "helpful tool in the decision-making process." However, "an inadequately prepared agenda can result in inadequate and unwise decisions" (ref. 20).

Agendas are the blueprints for meetings, defining directions for action. Serving as guidelines for general membership, board, or committee meetings, agendas define the structure upon which such meetings are built and indicate the directions in which the auxiliary is moving. Agendas are also guides to the writing of minutes, which, collectively, become a recording of the year's activities.

Conceived and utilized as a vehicle for advancing the auxiliary toward its goals, the agenda assumes the status of much more than a mere written presentation of the order of business. It establishes a profile of the auxiliary's major plans and problems, serving as a technique for focusing on the most urgent and important matters. As such, it can also serve as an impetus for action.

A carefully designed, comprehensive agenda, furnished to auxilians at the time that a meeting call is sent out, and accompanied by descriptive materials when necessary for clarification, can stimulate creative thinking in advance of the meeting, making the actual time spent *in* the meeting more productive. In addition, the agenda should be clear in its intent, explicitly stating the specific goals for that particular meeting. Without this overview, any meeting of the auxiliary can become a meaningless ritual.

It remains for the membership education committee, the auxiliary's president, and the committee chairmen to plan each agenda for its ability to fulfill these requirements — just as it is within their area of operation to determine whether or not reports should be included in programs for these meetings. The responsibility for planning agendas is divided in the following manner: the membership education committee and the auxiliary's president jointly devise the agenda for membership meetings; the president plans the agenda for board meetings; the committee chairman is the organizer for committee meetings.

A well-constructed agenda is characterized by good organization, selective inclusion of relevant subjects, and sufficient supplementary information on these subjects. All these qualities can make the agenda an informative tool of communication, with a value extending beyond the mere listing of the order of items in a meeting. Handled by leadership that is skillful in conducting meetings, such an agenda can make the difference between meetings that are productive and informative and those that are futile exercises.

Planning the agenda requires certain groundwork before its various elements can be properly assembled. The minutes of previous meetings should be studied to ensure that any unfinished business or matters that have been deferred to later meetings will be included. Auxiliary officers and committee chairmen should be consulted concerning possible inclusion of reports at board and membership meetings. For committee meetings, subcommittee chairmen should be extended this same courtesy by the committee chairmen.

The order of business that generally comprises the agenda is based upon parliamentary procedure in its simplest adaptation, derived from *Robert's Rules of Order, Newly Revised* (ref. 49). It consists of the reading of the minutes of the previous meeting (a formality that is usually avoided; instead, the minutes are approved by vote, as mentioned earlier) ; reports of officers and committee chairmen; reports or comments by staff of the insti- tution who may be present; unfinished and new business; an- nouncements; and adjournment. In addition, another category of business should be included covering *unforeseen* or *unknown new business,* in contrast to the type of new business that is known in advance of the meeting. This category can simply be denoted as "other new business," in order to differentiate it.

Items on the agenda should be described specifically if subject matter is to be effectively communicated. For example, when the agenda lists "reports of officers and committees," the description should detail, exactly, the topics and persons involved. This same procedure applies to "unfinished business," "new business," "an- nouncements," and other items. To the extent that such knowl- edge is available prior to the meeting, it should be expanded upon in the agenda. In designing a detailed, explanatory agenda, however, discretion should be exercised to ensure the provision of sufficient information without overtaxing the privilege. "A lengthy agenda, if well constructed, often means a short meet- ing" (ref. 62).

Language used in the agenda can also be helpful — and an obvious guide — in defining the responsibilities of those partici- pating in meetings. Action words such as *confirm, advise, approve, discuss,* and *decide* clearly delineate expectations in relation to subject matter.

The amount of time to be devoted to each topic on the agenda is an important consideration in any business meeting of the auxiliary. Responsibility for predetermining these time allot- ments, and for moving the meeting along, rests with the meet- ing's chairman. Prior to the event, she should loosely estimate the approximate time each topic will require, thereby arriving at a total running time for the meeting. It should be emphasized, however, that such time allotments are *tentative,* dependent upon the individual situation. Flexibility is necessary when attempting to adhere to a schedule, particularly when a meeting is being productive, with essential discussion running overtime. In this event, progress would be hindered by abrupt termination. If the chairman doesn't overload the agenda and thinks in terms of *approximate* time periods, she should be able to conduct meetings that accomplish their purposes without overtaxing participants.

Interim Financial Reports

Interim financial reports to the board, although similar in content to the yearly financial statements, are characterized by a greater immediacy, due to their more frequent issuance. Some auxiliary boards prefer monthly reports; others request bi-monthly or quarterly financial statements from their treasurers. Frequency is determined by the relevance of such reports to board planning. In addition to providing statistics on current asset value, revenue, and expenditures, the interim report is concerned with the near future — with upcoming projects that will be bringing in revenue and with the auxiliary's financial commitments to the institution that must be fulfilled within the next few months. This report attempts to predict potential changes in revenue sources and expenditure patterns that will affect the auxiliary's current and more immediate financial situation.

Committee Progress Reports

Of particular importance in determining the validity of presenting progress reports at membership or board meetings is each auxiliary's definition of the term "progress," discussed earlier. Unless a committee's activities have created a real change in a given situation, whether progressive or regressive, there is no justification for including that committee's report in the program for a membership meeting. Similarly, the auxiliary's board of directors should, appropriately, focus its attention on a committee report only (1) if the board needs to be informed about a significant stage of activity reached by that committee, (2) if a committee project requires initial approval and funding, or (3) if additional funding or decisions on operations are needed for an ongoing project. Communications with the board can be further enhanced if committee chairmen have been working closely with the president-elect and the vice presidents for service and community relations throughout the year, providing the foundation for reporting on committee activities.

In preparing their committee's reports for presentation at membership or board meetings, committee chairmen should ensure that such reports are "balanced, representing the thinking of the entire committee and not that of any individual, including the chairman. If the committee rubber-stamps the chairman's or anyone else's ideas, the report is built on shaky ground. Members won't work in support of such a report" (ref. 53).

Another aspect of the chairman's responsibility in preparing committee reports relates to decision making in the presence of a major division of opinion within the committee. If this occurs, "the chairman should allow and encourage minority reports. When the chairman makes a report, he should give, or have someone give, any minority views. In the absence of a minority representative, the chairman should frankly state that committee action was not unanimous, but that all agreed to be bound by the majority" (ref. 53).

Prior to meetings, the committee chairmen who are scheduled to make reports should provide for the distribution of a printed version to the general membership for its advance information. The auxiliary's newsletter can also be used as a vehicle for presenting a committee's views to the membership.

Notebooks

Other tools in the development of reports are the personal notebooks maintained by the auxiliary's president and committee chairmen. The president's notebook should contain pertinent facts on board decisions, the activities of each committee, and substantive information on meetings with the institution's chief executive. Committee notebooks are a running commentary on meetings held, decisions reached, assignments given, and projects undertaken. These notebooks provide a constant source of everyday reference. Collectively, the information they contain can be helpful in preparing the annual reports of the president and committee chairmen.

Another function of such notebooks is that they can be passed along from one year's leadership group to the next, providing valuable assistance to incoming officers and committee chairmen by alerting them to certain established events that require advance preparation. This profile of the previous year's activities gives successors a frame of reference for the handling of their own responsibilities.

Publicity and Related Materials

The auxiliary's community relations committee should assume the responsibility for maintaining a scrapbook of news clippings, photographs, and other materials relating to the auxiliary and the institution. In its assumption of this task, the committee will perform a job that has been traditionally handled, in many auxiliaries, by the historian. This manual suggests that the position of historian be eliminated and that the community relations committee be substituted, as a more contemporary approach to maintaining this type of material.

Retention of Records and Reports

The matter of retaining records and reports for specified periods must be determined by the individual auxiliary. Generally speaking, however, the auxiliary's annual reports, the treasurer's reports and financial statements, annual budgets, minutes from board and membership meetings, and bylaws and bylaws amendments are the documents that should be filed for permanent reference. Financial records, particularly, should be retained for a minimum of five years, and the institution's attorney may advise an even longer period. For historical purposes it may also be desirable to retain in the hospital's archives a selection from the other types of records mentioned. Of lesser importance but still to be considered for possible retention are the auxiliary's newsletters for the membership and reports to the community.

"These records must be on hand for review when it is time for evaluation of the auxiliary's programs and activities. Evaluation cannot be performed in a vacuum. A comparison of this year's records with those of preceding years is necessary to determine what progress has been made, what programs were successful, which goals have been reached and which remain" (ref. 53).

It is most important that a single repository be established for these records and reports, with one person responsible for receiving and retaining them. The auxiliary's secretary is the logical choice for this task, as discussed in the section on library resources in Chapter 8.

In pursuit of better communication, skillful recording and reporting can bring an auxiliary's total operation into focus for the membership, the institution, and the community. Motivating those responsible for the auxiliary's recording and reporting activities to develop skills in these important areas should be a primary obligation of leadership.

chapter 11
Planning and Evaluation

Planning is an orderly means used by an
organization to establish effective control over its
own future. . . . In some form, every organization
engages in planning, for without planning,
there would be little sense of purpose, direction,
or achievement. Planning provides the basis
for the work of the enterprise, and for evaluation of the
progress and effectiveness of that work.

Mrs. H. Lawrence Wilsey,
former member,
Committee on Volunteers,
American Hospital Association

Philosophy

To a considerable extent, the basic management of
the auxiliary — or of any organization — is dependent upon leadership's ability to use the planning and evaluation process to best
advantage. These interrelated functions are essential tools for
leadership in the effective and efficient management of the auxiliary's affairs. Well-conceived planning and evaluation practices
provide direction for the auxiliary and furnish opportunity to
thoroughly and systematically review and revise programs in the
interests of progress.

As an entity whose existence is based upon serving its institution and community, the auxiliary is obligated to plan and evaluate so as to provide this direction for progress. The result of

such a purposeful, analytical approach should be an effectively functioning auxiliary, capable of achieving its stated goals for its institution.

Planning and evaluation constitute one of the primary responsibilities of the auxiliary's leadership group, the board of directors. Together they encompass:

1. Reassessing the original purposes or goals of the auxiliary, for as the needs of the institution and the community change, the auxiliary may have to modify its purposes or goals accordingly.
2. Determining the specific objectives that represent a means of achieving the auxiliary's overall purposes or goals on behalf of the institution and the community.
3. Ascertaining where the responsibility for achieving these objectives should be assigned (committees, board of directors, officers).
4. Establishing criteria for assessing the effectiveness of the planning and evaluation process. This includes the ability to evaluate the validity of current objectives, once attained, as well as the efficacy of the methods used to reach these objectives.

Planning and evaluation are considered here as interrelated functions rather than two distinct activities because they are a continuum of the same process. This approach is best understood by visualizing planning and evaluation as an entire procedure, composed of a series of actions, each linked to the other and each dependent on the other for completion of the process. If leadership uses this interrelated approach to planning and evaluation in managing the immediate and long-range operations of the auxiliary, its programs should benefit considerably.

Planning and evaluation encompass a broad spectrum of functions and activities, ranging, for example, from the conceptual considerations involved in the creation of effective leadership development programs to improving the quality of the auxiliary's relationship with administration to the more concrete dollars and cents results of fund-raising projects and budgetary control.

Responsibility

In assuming the responsibility for the process of planning and evaluation, the board of directors holds the decisive key to the auxiliary's future, for it is through this process that an auxiliary's level of effectiveness is ultimately determined. The board must be able to envision near and distant goals, carry out the planning needed to achieve them, and recognize the importance of continual evaluation both as a means of assessing progress and as a method for propelling the auxiliary forward.

A realistic board should recognize that planning and evaluation demand in-depth deliberation, periodic brainstorming, and lengthy discussion. Accordingly, the board should provide for these time-consuming and comprehensive activities in its working schedule.

However, there may be times, particularly if new directions seem important, when the board may be unable to devote adequate attention to these essential activities. In such instances, the board, in the interests of practicality, may establish an ad hoc committee specifically charged with assessing the auxiliary's functions and, drawing upon this evaluation, recommending immediate and long-range plans for more effective operation. This planning committee could be authorized to function for a predetermined amount of time, with the board again assuming the responsibility at some point in the future. Or, such an ad hoc committee might eventually attain the status of a standing committee, should the board deem it necessary.

The planning committee could be composed of the auxiliary's president-elect and two vice presidents (service and community relations), in addition to regular members of the auxiliary, thereby providing input from the ranks of both leadership and general membership. Any such committee should have the benefit of input and feedback from the institution and other organizations that will be affected by the auxiliary's planning and subsequent activities. It is preferable to obtain this consultation by establishing an informal advisory relationship with appropriate representatives rather than by including them as members of the committee.

Whether the actual planning and evaluation activity is handled by the board of directors or by a committee, certain basic principles should be explored before initiating this process. Like the classic riddle of "Which came first, the chicken or the egg?", the planning process cannot proceed until the auxiliary's present programs and activities have first been evaluated. This implies recognizing the need to incorporate the evaluation procedure into the total planning process from the very beginning. Evaluation, in turn, relies upon the results of previous planning for its subject matter. Therefore, planning will be defined first and then the preparation for the planning process, which begins with evaluation, will be described.

What Is Planning?

The definition of planning quoted at the beginning of this chapter emphasizes the essential significance of planning to the overall management and functioning of the auxiliary. Another definition of planning is "an action-oriented process that encourages an institution to cope with change" (ref. 8). This definition is especially important to an auxiliary working on behalf of an institution that is attempting to meet the changing health care needs of its community in the most effective manner possible.

Robert M. Sigmond, executive vice president, Albert Einstein Medical Center, Philadelphia, offers the following definition: "Most simply stated, *planning is advance thinking as a basis for doing.* It is applied intelligence, an essential part of almost all human activity. But the planning that everyone does is usually extemporaneous and carried out with little attempt to be systematic and orderly. Most people and most organizations have analyzed neither the contents nor the effectiveness of their planning processes. . . . The issue, then, is not *whether* people do or should plan, but rather *how* planning can be improved and made a more useful activity" (ref. 7).

Drawing upon the substance of these definitions, planning can be described as an essential decision-making process that stimulates present action by an organization or institution in order to produce specific results at some future date. Planning should be a permanent, integral part of an organization's management processes and should lead ultimately to action, which is the logical goal of any planning effort.

Why Plan?

As an integral part of its institution, accountable to it, the auxiliary is obligated to plan for the most effective functioning it is capable of. Such an attitude about planning also justifies the trust, and the responsibility for performing certain functions, that the institution accords to the auxiliary.

This obligation to plan has other implications for the auxiliary. "Planning is a necessary tool to bring out and use the potential strength of a voluntary organization . . ." (ref. 44). It enables the auxiliary "to make the most efficient and effective use of the people and other resources available — a most desirable factor in attracting and keeping the able and enthusiastic members needed for carrying out a program" (ref. 44).

Another reason for planning is to provide continuity of operation. As the vehicle for the management of the auxiliary, each successive leadership group needs the motivation and momentum that solid planning makes possible from year to year in order to carry through programs and activities. "An auxiliary . . . must plan if it is to be successful, because with its periodic changes in leadership, it needs the continuity that results from the long-term view fostered by methodical planning" (ref. 44).

Planning is essential to an organization that depends on the public for moral and financial support and for potential auxilians or recruits for the institution's department of volunteer services. Projection of a positive image to this public is enhanced by an emphasis on serious and thoughtful planning. It demonstrates that the auxiliary is a group that knows where it is going and how to get there and that it intends to complete the trip by achieving its objectives.

A final and comprehensive viewpoint on the function of planning relates its value to accomplishments other than the development of the plans themselves. "There is logic behind the claim that the process of formal planning is perhaps just as useful as the results of planning. Indeed, one of the major benefits of a formal planning system is the fact that managers are required to put down on paper, in concrete terms, the informal plans which would otherwise guide their actions. In this fashion, they are forced to examine the present, learn from the past, and focus on the future. Glaring inconsistencies between stated goals and actual actions, or between different parts of the organization, are immediately brought to the surface, and corrective measures are adopted. Many such opportunities for improving current operations, if not discovered because of a formal planning effort, would be lost forever" (ref. 33).

When To Plan

Because the planning process, as conceived in this manual, is an in-depth and comprehensive procedure, short-range planning (the year ahead) and long-range planning should be conducted both annually and periodically, as the need arises. It would be preferable to begin the annual planning several months in advance of the end of the auxiliary's fiscal year and annual meeting. In this way, the auxiliary's annual report can reflect the past year's accomplishments (and failures), and can offer the auxiliary's projected plans for the next 12 months and beyond.

Planning will probably also be conducted spontaneously throughout the year, when individual situations develop that require immediate attention in terms of new strategic approaches, assignment of new responsibilities, or establishment of new committees.

There must be a correlation between the planning process and the budgeting process. The budget serves as a basic tool in planning programs and in setting program priorities and determines the financial feasibility of future operations. If evaluation indicates, for example, that more money will be required in the year ahead to expand the operation of successful programs, the auxiliary will be better able to provide for this in its new budget if it is fully aware of the needs *before* they occur. Similarly, evaluation may indicate that the auxiliary has been overinvesting funds in projects that can be operated more economically, thus freeing money for use in other programs. By planning for these contingencies in advance, the auxiliary is functioning effectively to meet future needs.

Long-Range Planning

Five years is generally considered to be a feasible unit of time for making long-range projections on the auxiliary's potential contributions in service and funds. Anything beyond this may fall into the category of speculation, unless the health care institution that the auxiliary serves has established a definitive plan of action for the next decade or longer.

An amusing quotation perhaps sums up the eternal question: "How long is long-range?" According to Joseph P. Peters, former associate executive director, Health and Hospital Planning Council of Southern New York, Inc.: "There have been numerous attempts to develop a meaningful time period that constitutes long-range. I am told that pulp and paper companies claim to prepare plans on a 40-year basis. Companies producing products subject to rapid style changes consider anything beyond a year or two as irrelevant. Many industries — and nations — have settled on five years as their long-range planning period. Why five years? The former director of planning at IBM gives perhaps the most reasonable explanation for this choice. 'We chose five years,' he said, 'because four years are too short and six years are too long' " (ref. 8).

Long-range plans should be reviewed at least annually, and revised if necessary. They should be flexible in design (as should plans for the immediate future), so that revision is possible without having to conduct a major overhaul. Such plans "should provide guidelines that are firm enough to give direction, but not so rigid as to limit the possibilities for action, or to stifle the creative approach oncoming auxiliary members may have" (ref. 65). In addition, such plans should be comprehensive, encompassing all the auxiliary's programs and services.

Those responsible for planning should be thinking in terms of the auxiliary's potential contributions in service, funds, and time. They should ask questions that will help define the needs of the institution and the community, and use the answers to shape their long-range and immediate programs for the auxiliary. Utilizing this approach, plans will be logical, in agreement with the institution's goals or objectives.

As a contemporary example of long-range planning, one of the auxiliary's major objectives might be to assist its institution in providing care for the nonacute patient who can be maintained outside the hospital. Those responsible for implementing this particular objective might determine that it could best be achieved through provision of some of the following services: meals for shut-ins or convalescing patients, visiting nurse and homemaker programs, and "telecare" (for example, telephone communication between an auxilian and a posthospital patient during the first few weeks after the patient returns home). The auxiliary could provide financing for all of these services and staffing for some of them. These services, all of which represent methods of attaining the desired objective, constitute the action phase of long-range planning.

Before selecting the appropriate methods for accomplishing this objective, the committee responsible for this program would have to consider the feasibility of implementing each of the various services. Matters for consideration, prior to making any commitment to conduct specific activities, would include budget, the auxiliary's personnel who would be available to participate in the program, motivation and education of membership, community education, and the attitudes of related community agencies.

Evaluation

The process of planning and evaluation is cyclical. The planning function cannot begin until the auxiliary's present situation has been thoroughly and objectively evaluated. The results of this assessment provide the basis for the actual planning activity. It becomes evident, then, that the planning function itself requires planning or preparation and that evaluation is the initial step.

Evaluation can be considered as a normal process of progress. It is the tool that facilitates measurement of the effectiveness of current programs and activities in relation to previously established standards of performance. Without evaluation, planning would be conducted in limbo, with no previous experience to use as a frame of reference.

"As the practice of evaluating performance continues over the years, the auxiliary acquires a valuable record of experience and methods that can act as a guide in future planning — not only for what has proved successful, but for what has not. Applied to current action, evaluation can also indicate the need for modification or revision, before it is too late. This is desirable, both from the point of view of efficiency, and to maintain the morale of the members and the prestige of the auxiliary. However, in accumulating experience, we must remember that we must be selective about what we accept, and that what is good at one time may become outmoded or inappropriate at another. Experience itself counts for little. It is what our critical judgment makes of it that enables us to progress" (ref. 44).

From the viewpoint of organizational management, evaluation is an asset for unifying and strengthening an auxiliary by focusing the members' attention on achievement. Evaluation is a means for maintaining the interest of those involved by "restating the goals, and reminding us that something is being done. Furthermore, it is an excellent method of giving practical experience and training to potential leaders" (ref. 44).

In terms of the planning of the auxiliary's affairs for the next year or longer, the evaluation function is, virtually, a "postmortem" analysis of the results of last year's planning (or the last five years, depending upon the span of time used by the planning group). The evaluation function, however, has applications beyond the yearly review of the auxiliary's performance. It should also be a built-in function of every ongoing program and activity conducted by the auxiliary throughout the year. If it is considered a continuing function, utilized on an everyday basis as well as annually, it becomes an intrinsic part of the auxiliary's total planning process. Operating in this way, evaluation can be used to continually update, revise, and review the auxiliary's plans, even as they are being implemented, if necessary. "A point not to be missed here is that continual evaluation permits early (and therefore usually more easily accomplished) corrective action . . . the means for evaluation [should] be decided upon when an activity or program is first planned, making it easier to see whether the program is evolving as planned" (ref. 64).

If the auxiliary is newly organized, it cannot, of course, draw upon its evaluation of past experience in order to plan ahead — unless it had an unfortunate predecessor! However, the very process of analyzing the possibility of an auxiliary's serving a specific institution with certain needs, within a given community, is, in itself, evaluative in nature, as described in Chapter 12, "How To Start an Auxiliary."

The following steps in evaluating the auxiliary's programs and performance are important during the preplanning stage:

1. Determine areas for evaluation.
2. Obtain data on these subjects.
3. Compare present data to previous expectations for achievement (as expressed in planning), to determine whether the auxiliary's current levels of performance are acceptable. Results of this analysis should also show whether the auxiliary has established and is maintaining realistic standards of performance against which the auxiliary's implementa-

tion of programs can be measured, and whether the programs themselves are still valid.

4. On the basis of this information, determine areas of the auxiliary's operations that deserve priority in planning.

Overall Goals

The auxiliary's board of directors assumes the responsibility for establishing and periodically reassessing the broad goals or purposes of the auxiliary. These goals can be articulated in general terms, such as "helping the institution to provide better and more comprehensive health care to the community" or "providing the funds and services to assist the institution in functioning more effectively as a provider of health care."

The overall goals or purposes of the auxiliary are somewhat more permanent than its objectives, which may fluctuate according to the institution's current approach to accommodating the community's health care needs. Nevertheless, when determining appropriate goals for itself, the auxiliary should take into consideration various factors and the possibility that these may change. The institution's requirements are a primary factor. These will be based on the community's health care needs and its perception of these needs. The auxiliary also should consider such factors as the composition of the community, each auxilian's concept of the auxiliary's central purposes, and the attitudes of other volunteer groups related to health care toward their roles in the community.

"To establish the purpose of an auxiliary, it is necessary that the expectations of the hospital, the auxilians, other voluntary bodies, and the community be kept under constant review, for they will change, and purposes must change with them. A leader's role in this key activity is not to identify purpose in isolation, but to involve as many people as possible in the process. In this way, more information will be made available and more commitment ensured" (ref. 63).

Unless the auxiliary's conception of its basic purposes corresponds to the real needs of the institution and the community, it cannot serve effectively. This becomes readily apparent all the way down the line, with objectives being poorly articulated and programs failing to produce results that are realistically desirable. An open channel of communication between the auxiliary's president and the institution's chief executive and governing board, and between the auxiliary's leadership and appropriate community representatives, can help to ensure that the determination of the objectives and of the programs that are the means for attaining these goals is rooted in realism.

Specific Objectives

An objective is the desired result of a proposed plan of action or change in a situation. A statement of objectives should denote measurable qualities observable by the auxiliary's leadership; otherwise it is impossible to determine whether programs meet objectives.

Responsibility for evaluating the validity of the auxiliary's objectives, and the effectiveness of the programs and activities that have been used as a vehicle for achieving them, can be assumed by either the board of directors or a planning committee. Whatever the situation, those engaged in the planning and evaluation process would be advised to query themselves as to what the auxiliary is doing, why the auxiliary is doing it, how the auxiliary is doing it, and how the auxiliary can do it better. Areas for the application of these questions, within the sphere of the auxiliary's current operations, could include the following:

- **Organization and management.** Concerning the auxiliary's overall performance, did the auxiliary reach its objectives as defined within the past year to five years? If not, was this because the objectives were not feasible or appropriate in terms of meeting the institution's or the community's needs? Were the methods for achieving these objectives (programs, projects, activities) poorly conceived and therefore doomed to failure? Were other methods available that would have been more effective, less costly, easier? If objectives *were* reached, what were the strengths inherent in the methods used or in the objectives themselves? How well have the planning and evaluation functions worked in terms of results achieved throughout the year? What types of programs and projects should the auxiliary be developing to better and more realistically serve the institution and the community?

- **Outside influences.** Are the developments arising out of local and regional health care planning affecting the institution in its provision of health care services, which, in turn, influence the auxiliary in its program planning? What is the effect of new federal laws concerning the provision of health care? Can the changes emanating from all these sources be accommodated by the auxiliary in its planning and performance?

- **Community relations.** In what ways has community reaction influenced the success or failure of the auxiliary's programs and projects? If such reaction has been negative, was it because leadership incorrectly assessed the possible response, or did unforeseen circumstances create problems? Have community representatives been requested to contribute evaluations of the auxiliary's programs? What are the effects on the auxiliary of the programs and activities conducted by other health care institutions and agencies within the community at large and the auxiliaries serving these institutions? Are the auxiliary's fund-raising efforts meeting with success in the community, in terms of being a vehicle for improving human relations? Or is the auxiliary wearing out its proverbial welcome with too frequent, unskilled solicitation, events, and so forth.

- **Membership relations.** How is membership participation affecting the success or failure of the auxiliary's programs? Is the general membership being sufficiently involved in the planning and decision-making processes to motivate its support? How is the auxiliary's membership education program contributing to this motivation? Is it comprehensive, providing information about ongoing and projected programs, or is it merely a token effort, giving only superficial orientation about the auxiliary's affairs? What are the figures for the past year regarding meeting attendance, membership recruitment, and membership retention? Can committee chairmen honestly report that committee members have responded enthusiastically to their assignments and been productive in carrying them out?

- **Leadership development.** How has the auxiliary's leadership development program affected the attainment of objectives?

Has it created an effective leadership group, capable of achieving objectives within the committee and board structures? If not, is the reason attributable to a lack of continuity in leadership training from one year to the next, indicating poor planning? Or has such training simply been underdeveloped, static, and not sufficiently purposeful? Does the leadership group regularly engage in self-evaluation, measuring its own performance against certain predetermined standards to ascertain its sufficiency? For example, how effective is the board in meeting problems? Do committee chairmen evaluate the performance of their committees, in addition to the evaluation conducted by the board? Does each chairman also assess her own capabilities?

• **Relationship with the institution.** What is the nature of the relationship between the auxiliary's leadership and the institution's chief executive and governing board? If there are problems, can they be attributed to lack of communication, misinterpretation of the auxiliary's objectives, or misunderstanding about the auxiliary's appropriate place in the structure of authority existing among the three entities? Are the programs of the auxiliary keeping pace with the institution's present and projected needs? If not, is this due to a communications gap between the administration and the auxiliary's leadership, or is leadership, itself, somehow not acknowledging the need for change in attitudes and approaches to the auxiliary's programs? Is the auxiliary's relationship with the institution's professional staff and employees creating goodwill and better understanding, so that the auxiliary can function optimally? Have the institution's representatives, at various professional levels, been asked to informally evaluate the auxiliary's programs?

• **Fund raising and financial affairs.** Is the auxiliary's current fund-raising program meeting realistic financial goals? If it is falling short, are the reasons related to the techniques involved in fund raising; the skills of the individuals involved in conducting fund-raising functions, whether direct solicitation or events; the availability of manpower to staff projects; uses for the funds, which may be misdirected or miscalculated; or the auxiliary's budgetary planning and implementation? Is the auxiliary's concept of budgeting realistic, in terms of its actual needs and those of its institution? Are capable individuals serving on the finance committee? Is the treasurer functioning effectively?

Data Gathering

The two primary sources of data for the planning and evaluation process are verbal feedback and records and reports.

Verbal Feedback

Feedback tells an organization where it is in terms of accomplishment, unmet needs, and progress. It provides a tool for evaluating the situation and determining which elements are needed to make programs successful.

An obvious starting place for the generation of information would be discussions between the auxiliary's board of directors or planning committee and the auxiliary's committee chairmen. At some point, the general membership should be brought into the assessment process. This is particularly important if the board, rather than the planning committee, is doing the planning for the auxiliary and has no representation or input from the general membership. Feedback from community representatives, as described earlier, should also be incorporated into the data-gathering process, if the auxiliary is to develop a broad and realistic frame of reference for its program planning.

Other channels of communication with the institution should be used in addition to those already mentioned between the auxiliary's president, the institution's chief executive, and the governing board. Where auxiliary committees have counterparts within the institution's structure, there is fertile opportunity for obtaining information that may be helpful in evaluating the auxiliary's present operations. As described in Chapter 8, "Education," a correlation of functions and sharing of objectives does exist in the areas of community relations-public relations, financial affairs, volunteer services, and perhaps others.

An example of a sharing of objectives is the relationship between the auxiliary's scholarship committee and the institution's personnel department. The director of personnel would be concerned with the provision of continuing education programs for the institution's employees and the promotion of new types of careers in the health care field. If these needs are communicated to the scholarship committee by the personnel director, the auxiliary can ensure that its advance planning includes provisions for financial assistance for deserving employees and a continuing effort to recruit health career oriented persons into the field. A similar sharing of objectives would require that the auxiliary's community relations committee work in concert with the appropriate personnel within the institution to promote patient and community health education.

Discussion among the auxiliary's board, committees, and membership, person-to-person interviews with community and institutional representatives, and unsolicited comments offered by individuals during the course of the year can all provide substance for the information-gathering procedure. "An accurate evaluation will be a synthesis of the estimates made, not only by those directing the program and those involved in implementing it, but will take into account the impressions of those affected by the program, and of general opinion" (ref. 44). Expression of many viewpoints is necessary if the broad spectrum of questions concerning the auxiliary's objectives is to be adequately and correctly answered.

Records and Reports

The other major sources of information in this evaluation process are the auxiliary's records and reports for the past five years, with particular emphasis on the year just passed. A close examination of these documents by the auxiliary's leadership should disclose any variance between expectations and actual accomplishments in the achievement of the central objectives that the auxiliary had established for itself. This variance will be most easily measurable in such areas as membership interest, as expressed by retention of members and meeting attendance, and community support of the auxiliary's activities, as evidenced by attendance at auxiliary-sponsored events, interest in joining the auxiliary or the institution's department of volunteer services, and the amount and number of financial contributions.

The quotation by Mrs. Harry Milton in Chapter 10, "Records and Reports," given in the section concerning the importance of retaining these documents, deserves repeating:

"These records must be on hand for review when it is time for evaluation of the auxiliary's programs and activities. Evaluation cannot be performed in a vacuum. A comparison of this year's records with those of preceding years is necessary to determine what progress has been made, what programs were successful, which goals have been reached and which remain" (ref. 40). In discussing the value of records and reports to evaluation, Mrs. Milton comments on the significance of what has gone before to what will come. Her attitude suggests that planning ahead cannot be a valid process until past efforts have been examined and that utilization of records and reports is a means to this end.

As an input to evaluation, records and reports should provide a comprehensive view of past planning efforts, including (1) why specific plans (objectives and methods) were adopted, (2) the success or failure of those plans, and the reasons involved, leading logically to (3) why certain changes were made.

If records and reports *don't* furnish this type of information, it is suggested that the auxiliary specifically evaluate its recording and reporting processes, along the lines described in Chapter 10. Thus, examination of records and reports, in addition to guiding the auxiliary in its evaluation efforts, can also indicate the need to strengthen other processes.

Feedback from within and outside of the auxiliary, combined with the data provided by records and reports, should bring the auxiliary's planning group to the next stage in evaluation. This would be the comparison of the auxiliary's expectations for achievement, as reflected in previous planning, to the actual accomplishments of the auxiliary in relation to these plans. From this comparison, levels of performance are shown.

Standards of Performance

"Establishing criteria with which to measure or appraise a program is fundamental to the evaluation of results. Deciding upon criteria should be an integral part of the planning process for any activity" (ref. 23).

Each auxiliary has its own criteria for what constitutes adequate, superior, and inferior performance. These criteria are based upon the auxiliary's past experience in achieving objectives, contrasted with its present capabilities. If previous plans were carefully formulated, and articulated in specific terms, it should not be difficult to identify problem or success producing areas relating to choice of objectives, or the programs and activities that represent a means of attaining them. Disparities between planning and achievement should become apparent, as will the attainment or surpassing of goals. "An auxiliary should not attempt to evaluate only the portion of its program that it believes is in trouble, nor to analyze only a particular activity that has been successful, but should include both the good and the bad" (ref. 64).

If an auxiliary has difficulty in reaching conclusions with this basic type of comparison process, the problem may be that objectives were not sufficiently well defined to provide some criteria for measuring the progress or success of programs. Without clearly stated objectives that are understood by the auxiliary, and somehow measurable, it is impossible to evaluate programs efficiently. Further, there is no sound basis for selecting the best methods for achieving these objectives.

When there is considerable variance between expectations for performance — as expressed in previous plans — and current levels of achievement, it is possible that standards of performance are unrealistic. Here, the auxiliary has established a situation in which it is attempting to accomplish objectives that are just not feasible for this particular group. The reasons might be related to insufficient manpower, lack of membership motivation, inadequate funding for operation of projects, weak and indecisive leadership, unclear objectives, or negative community response.

Another possibility is that the auxiliary is using improper methods (programs, activities) to achieve objectives. This can mean that the programs themselves are no longer valid in terms of the institution's or community's needs because a major shift has occurred in emphasis or priorities on the immediate health care scene or that the techniques used by auxilians to implement these programs may be incorrect in approach, coming across as too aggressive, repetitive, unimaginative, or purposeless.

"An evaluation is a guide, but not in itself a solution; its purpose is not fulfilled until conclusions are drawn" (ref. 44). And, one might add, "until remedial action is taken." It is not sufficient for the auxiliary to identify the reasons for the success or failure of its programs. Rather, it should go a step further and take appropriate action to change or correct situations when necessary.

Priorities for Planning

The status of the auxiliary's operations, its successes and failures, should become evident through the process of comparison. When the auxiliary has established where it is, compared to where it was, it is ready to determine which areas of operation deserve inclusion in the planning process for the immediate year ahead and which should be slated for long-range consideration. In other words, evaluation should show need.

Perhaps examination discloses that there is a single, major aspect of the auxiliary's functions that requires an overhaul, such as its total approach to fund raising. If this is the case, the fund-raising program would receive primary emphasis in the auxiliary's planning efforts. Or there may be a number of possible areas that require change and whose objectives or programs require close review and revision. In this latter situation, however, it is not practicable or desirable for an auxiliary to attempt an overly ambitious program of major change. "For this reason, an auxiliary finds it necessary to assign priorities to possible projects, assessing them on the basis of importance, need, precedence, cost, and feasibility. This is one instance where the quality of leadership is tested; it is not always easy to determine what is more important or more needed. It requires vision and courage sometimes to put first things first" (ref. 44).

The objectives that will form the substance for the planning process "must be chosen on the basis of their place in the hierarchy of need, and the availability of group resources. As objectives are formulated, care should be taken to ensure that they are totally understandable; compatible with resources . . . needs and expectations; and measurable" (ref. 63).

Being aware of what gives certain objectives priority over others will help an auxiliary to make its planning meaningful. It will be based upon a recognition of what the auxiliary really needs to be doing, as well as what it *can* do.

Proper evaluation techniques thus play an important role in the stage prior to actual planning. By feeding the necessary kind of information into the planning process through these specific evaluation procedures, the auxiliary has already achieved the first step toward successful planning and implementation. Without the correct input from evaluation, planning becomes an exercise in futility. Poorly assessed priorities, misconceived objectives, and erroneous methods of conducting programs can become entrenched in practice and perpetuated from year to year.

"If we expect evaluation to help us discover the problems with our programs and to set realistic sights about how much we can accomplish for people, then it is an effective tool. It does have purpose and worth, and is especially vital in policy setting, planning, and administration" (ref. 25).

Putting Action into Planning

In initiating the actual planning process, action must be put into planning before plans can be put into action! When the planning group has reached agreement on those objectives that carry priority status for the auxiliary, it should be in a position to proceed with the creation of immediate and long-range plans. This can encompass a series of actions including: correction of undesirable and unproductive situations through change in concept, approach, or personnel; continuation of successful programs; or initiation of entirely new programs and activities to meet present needs or to anticipate future needs.

The process of *planning by objectives,* once they are established, leads to the next logical step, *planning for action or implementation.* This involves indicating the broad areas of activity that will most successfully resolve the problems facing the auxiliary and help it to obtain or maintain specific, desired results in the various areas of its operations. It also entails designation of the groups or individuals within the auxiliary's organizational structure that will be responsible for implementing these plans.

Taking into consideration the auxiliary's capabilities and limitations, as determined through the evaluation process, the planning group should provide answers to the following questions in order to organize its plan for action:

* What are the actual steps involved, and what will be the forms of action or organization necessary to implement them?
* What will be the length of time needed to reach such objectives? (This involves the setting of target dates, if possible.) Should a detailed schedule be followed in executing plans?

- How much will specific programs cost? Although the planning group may have to be approximate in its estimation, it should attempt to come as close to actual figures as possible. This is essential for the establishment of budget requests and proper provision of funds.
- Are possible alternatives to programs or activities available, should they be needed?
- Will the auxiliary's present internal education and communications techniques be effective in getting programs and related responsibilities across to the membership and in coordinating efforts?
- Will specific programs duplicate other ongoing endeavors of the auxiliary or previous work? Will they duplicate efforts of other auxiliaries or health care agencies in the community?
- What are the strengths and weaknesses of the auxiliary's organizational structure, which is the basis for any action program? Will specific committees and individuals be able to accomplish desired objectives?
- Does the auxiliary know the specific skills required to attain these objectives, in terms of human effort?
- Who will be responsible for handling specific tasks?
- What is the availability of resources in terms of the auxiliary's manpower, variety of talent, and financial support?
- Will certain programs and activities require the participation of the institution or community groups in order to be implemented?
- Do the more immediate, short-range programs and activities build toward the long-range plans of the auxiliary?

The responses to these questions should provide the structure upon which plans can be created. When plans are articulated in written form, they should be comprehensive and detailed, clearly indicating their scope and defining the broad areas of responsibilities and relationships of those who will be carrying out the plans. However, the planning group should avoid being *too* specific regarding the ways in which committees will meet the charges for action given to them.

If a committee receives a charge for the implementation of activities, it also deserves to be granted latitude in developing the methods it will use to fulfill its assignment. This means that a committee creates its own plan of action in response to a charge. Such an approach helps a committee to expand its scope of performance and to utilize its imaginative and creative abilities. It also can test the leadership capacities of the committee chairman and can stimulate the development of leadership qualities in committee members.

Prior to the actual assignment of responsibilities and implementation, the board of directors should submit the plans to the institution's chief executive, and to the general membership, for final approval. This procedure is described in Chapter 5, "Committees," in the section entitled "Action Programs."

The planning group and committee chairmen should be acutely aware of this principle: "In organizing your human and physical resources, bear in mind at all times the balance between what you plan to do, and the people and facilities available to you" (ref. 57). This awareness leads to the development of realistic expectations for performance.

Putting Planning into Action

Translating plans into action is the next stage of leadership's responsibility. However, it is not always a straightforward trip. Plans often must change to adapt to changing circumstances. "A plan is a poor one indeed if it precludes modification. Flexibility is one of the absolute necessities of a workable plan. We have been led to believe that mistakes are a sign of weakness, when in truth they are the price of true learning. Each plan must have a face-saving mechanism built into it which will permit revision, or even rejection, without embarrassment to those who have contributed time and effort to its formulation. The absence of a face-saving device is a defect which can seriously handicap an honest search for a constructive course of action" (ref. 21).

If leadership is flexible in its implementation of plans, and the plans themselves can accommodate change, the auxiliary should realize a higher proportion of success in the action phase of its efforts and in reaching its ultimate objectives and goals.

Completing the Cycle

When the auxiliary has implemented its major plans for the year, the planning group returns to the evaluation process, coming full circle to the point from which it began. In addition to using the evaluation process to develop new plans, as described earlier, the planning group will also want to assess the effectiveness of the previous planning and evaluation procedures as entities unto themselves. The auxiliary's current status in relation to its objectives depends heavily upon the planning group's ability to accurately evaluate situations and to incorporate its conclusions into plans. Unless the planning and evaluation procedures are thoroughly analyzed — and this chapter suggests the qualities that these procedures should possess — it may be difficult to realistically determine a direction for the auxiliary, or to achieve desired objectives.

"Auxiliary leaders who pursue a formal program planning process will be amazed to discover how much an auxiliary can do, what varied programs it can undertake, and how hard the members will work to reach tangible, understood goals" (ref. 36).

chapter 12
How To Start an Auxiliary

The question of how best to serve the needs of a health care institution through volunteer participation is a highly individualized matter. Each institution and the community it serves have specialized needs that an auxiliary may or may not be able to fulfill.

Admittedly, the number of auxiliaries throughout the country bears testimony to the effectiveness and value of their work for health care institutions. However, this fact should not obscure the need for an organizing group to confront the basic issue of whether an auxiliary is actually wanted or needed in *its* community.

Within any given institution and its community, a diversity of situations may exist that have direct bearing on the need to establish an auxiliary. The institution's department of volunteer services, for example, may function sufficiently well to make an auxiliary seem unnecessary. The prevailing attitude may not recognize the added contributions an auxiliary can make. Conversely, this same department may be unsuccessfully attempting to cope with increasing demands for volunteer services and would welcome the help of an auxiliary. In an institution without such a department, an auxiliary may be urgently needed to assume the responsibilities that the department would normally handle.

In further assessing the need for an auxiliary, an organizing group should also consider the state of the institution's relationship to the community. Is there a definite need for better communication between the two entities, a function that an auxiliary could help serve? (See Chapter 5, "Committees.") Can an auxiliary, through its own representative membership and its personal contacts with individuals and organizations, suggest what the community wants and needs in health education and services? Would such an auxiliary be capable of providing the volunteer manpower to staff projects that would help meet these needs?

A realistic analysis of all these variables must occur before an auxiliary can assume its role as an effective volunteer organization, able to serve its institution and community in the most productive way. Whether the idea for an auxiliary is advanced by the institution's chief executive officer, members of the governing board, individuals connected with the institution in other capacities, or individuals within the community who recognize the possible need, all these persons must get together on the essentials regarding the establishment of the auxiliary and develop a clear and honest concept of their goals.

It is essential to develop a solid rationale on the advantages of having an auxiliary, illustrating how such an organization can help to expand the present services of its institution and increase its responsiveness to the health care needs of the community. Both the American Hospital Association and the appropriate state hospital association can be most helpful to an organizing group in developing criteria for the establishment of an auxiliary and can contribute to the presentation that will be made to the appropriate individuals when the subject is opened for discussion.

Assuming that the initiators of the auxiliary are community representatives who have reached the conviction that an auxiliary can perform a viable function, the next move would be to arrange a meeting between the institution's chief executive officer and the organizing group. In preparation for this gathering, the community representatives should develop a well-defined, concise, and persuasive presentation of their plan. To make their own convictions contagious, they will have to persuade the chief executive officer, and through him the governing board, that such an organization is truly needed: to make the auxiliary a working reality, they will have to gain a commitment of support.

Once there is general agreement on the goals of the auxiliary and the initial projects that will be conducted, the official approval of the chief executive officer and the board should be verified. From this point, arrangements can be made to enlarge the scope of planning by (1) obtaining the reactions of key individuals in the community and (2) holding a mass meeting of the community in order to recruit auxiliary members.

This initial meeting of key persons, numbering from 20 to 50 participants, should be representative of the entire community. Some of these individuals will be related to the health field; others, to community agencies and organizations. The chief executive officer and the organizing group can draw these participants from their personal and professional contacts. Among its participants, the meeting should include a member of the governing board, the chief executive officer, and, if desired, a member of the medical staff.

It may be helpful to invite an individual who is thoroughly familiar with auxiliaries to serve as a consultant on the problems of organization. Such a resource person could be a state auxiliary leader, a staff member from the state hospital association, or a representative from the American Hospital Association. By making use of this individual's expertise and knowledge of the total auxiliary picture, the organizing group can obtain a more comprehensive understanding of its efforts.

This meeting will still be a preliminary exercise, exploratory in nature, at which the organizing group, with the institution's approval, can present the agreed-upon concepts of the auxiliary's total role. A broad spectrum of cross-community viewpoints will be sought on the establishment of such an organization. Through this give-and-take a concrete decision should emerge.

If the majority agrees that an auxiliary should be created, a temporary chairman and committee should be authorized and appointed by the institution, including its attorney as one of the members. This committee will be entrusted with establishing a legal form for the auxiliary and writing bylaws.

In addition to handling the legal and organizational details, the committee will also need to prepare for the presentation of its plans to the community at large. Because acceptance of the auxiliary and membership recruitment are the motivating factors for this projected mass meeting, a printed promotional piece highlighting the auxiliary's proposed objectives and projects should be created by the committee and distributed, along with copies of the proposed bylaws, at the meeting.

Attendance can be stimulated by having the committee work in tandem with the institution's public relations-community relations department, which can provide the appropriate media and organizational contacts. If such a department does not exist, the committee, with the approval of the chief executive officer, can develop its own channels of communication and implement the advance publicity.

During the meeting, membership should be actively solicited. Later, at the first membership meeting, bylaws will be adopted, officers elected, and orientation begun.

It is hoped that this manual, with its in-depth treatment of subjects that are significant to auxiliaries, will serve as a continuing frame of reference for the organizing group. From the inception and initial development of the auxiliary, through its years of growth, this book can truly be used as a working manual.

appendix A
Model Bylaws

The following model bylaws have been prepared for the guidance of an auxiliary that is legally established as an integral part of a voluntary not-for-profit health care institution. With appropriate substitution for the word *hospital*, which is used throughout, these bylaws can also serve as a model to guide an auxiliary established as an integral part of any health care institution. Furthermore, with some changes in language, they can be adapted to the needs of an incorporated auxiliary or an auxiliary that is an unincorporated association.

These model bylaws should not be adopted verbatim. They must be adapted to fit particular local conditions and needs. Where the auxiliary is functioning in a health care institution other than the voluntary type — such as investor-owned or government — special consideration must be exercised in adapting the model bylaws to individual use.

In determining the most appropriate organizational form and in preparing bylaws, an auxiliary should always seek and follow the advice of the institution's attorney.

ARTICLE I. NAME
The name of this organization shall be   (name of institution) Auxiliary or the Auxiliary of   (name of institution).

Comment
    Although other names are used, the suggested name has several advantages: (1) it publicizes and emphasizes the hospital;

(2) the term *hospital auxiliary* is most commonly used and therefore best understood; (3) the definitions of *auxiliary* — conferring help, supporting, subsidiary, serving to supplement — describe precisely the purpose of a community group dedicated to the service of its hospital; (4) the exclusion of a gender prefix (such as *women's*) indicates that the auxiliary is truly a community organization, open to men as well as women interested in the hospital.

ARTICLE II. PURPOSE

The purpose of this organization shall be to render service to (name of institution) and its patients and to assist (name of institution) in promoting the health and welfare of the community in accordance with objectives established by the institution.

Comment

The suggested statement of purpose is succinct and, at the same time, covers two essential points: (1) it gives the fundamental reason for the auxiliary's existence and (2) it recognizes the ultimate authority of the institution. Such a simple yet all-encompassing statement serves also to differentiate between the broad goal of the auxiliary and the specific functions the auxiliary may be authorized to undertake in accomplishing its stated goal. Although not improper, further elaboration may tend to obscure the purpose of the auxiliary and to focus attention on means rather than ends.

ARTICLE III. MEMBERSHIP

Section 1. Membership in the auxiliary shall be open to all adults who are interested in (name of institution) and willing to uphold the purpose of the auxiliary. Membership shall become effective when the signed application for membership is received by the membership relations committee, on behalf of the auxiliary, and when the initial dues are paid.

Comment

Today's hospital seeks and receives support, moral and financial, from all segments of the community. It follows, therefore, that membership in the community organization affiliated with and dedicated to the welfare of the hospital should be open to all interested adults, regardless of race, religion, or social position. The term *adult* excludes persons under 18 (and in some states, under 21), but further interpretation of the term is left to the individual auxiliary and its institution.

The act of membership represents, in essence, a responsible commitment on the part of the individual to the purpose of the auxiliary and acceptance by the auxiliary of the individual's commitment. This act takes the form of an agreement when the prospective member applies formally, acknowledging willingness to uphold the purpose and the policies of the auxiliary and to abide by its bylaws, and when the membership relations committee, acting for the auxiliary membership, accepts the application. The initial agreement is renewed automatically by the annual payment and acceptance of dues.

Section 2. Members are in good standing as long as they uphold the agreement stated in the application for membership and renew their dues annually.

Section 3. Only members in good standing for_____ month(s) shall have the right to vote and to hold office in the auxiliary.

Section 4. A member may resign by submitting a written resignation to the auxiliary. The resignation shall be effective upon its acceptance by the board of directors, which shall be authorized to waive any delinquent dues or other indebtedness of the member.

Comment

A member may be required to pay delinquent dues or other indebtedness before her resignation will be accepted, but the board of directors may choose to waive the debts if the resignation is in the best interests of the auxiliary.

Section 5. Discretion to renew or refuse to renew a membership lies with the board of directors of the auxiliary. Refusal to renew shall be dependent on written notice being given to the member affected, with an opportunity within_____ days of such notice to make written request for a hearing on the refusal.

Comment

This arrangement allows for a simple and unemotional method of terminating the membership of individuals who, because they have failed to uphold the agreement under which they became members or for other reasons, are no longer an asset to the auxiliary. The board should be certain that it has

adequate justification for such action, even though there may
be no request for giving the dropped member a hearing.

Section 6. The auxiliary may confer honorary membership on
an individual in recognition of outstanding service to the auxiliary, the hospital, or the community. An honorary member shall
have no right to vote, unless the honorary member is also a
member in good standing as defined in Section 2 of this article.

Comment

Honorary membership offers to the auxiliary a means of
recognizing unusual service by an individual. It is and should
be used sparingly. There should be an established procedure
for nominating persons to receive honorary memberships.
Such nominations are subject to approval by the membership
at any regular meeting.

A further differentiation of membership into active and
inactive members, or regular and sustaining (or associate)
members, is not recommended.

ARTICLE IV. DUES

Section 1. Membership dues shall be $_____a year,
billed by and payable to the treasurer within the first month
of the fiscal year, which begins (day and month) and ends
(day and month).

Comment

Membership dues should be kept moderate, but the total
should be adequate to underwrite the auxiliary's basic operating expenses.

Section 2. Any dues owing on _____ of each year
shall be delinquent. Such nonpayment of dues shall automatically
suspend the membership, irrespective of notice. Reinstatement
shall be permitted upon approval of an application submitted to
the auxiliary's board of directors and payment of dues for the
current year.

Section 3. Dues and other payments made to the auxiliary
by members shall not be subject to refund, and the members shall
have no further individual rights to such funds.

Comment

As a result of this provision a member who resigns or
whose membership is terminated will have no right to a refund
of dues or fees previously paid.

Section 4. Honorary members shall not be required to pay dues.

Comment
> See Article III, Section 6.

ARTICLE V. MEETINGS OF THE AUXILIARY

Section 1. The auxiliary membership shall meet in regular session at least _____times a year, in addition to the annual meeting.

Section 2. The time and place of the meetings shall be determined by the president and/or the board of directors. Notice of any special meeting of the auxiliary membership shall be mailed to the members not less than 10 days in advance of such meeting.

Comment
> Where facilities are suitable, it is recommended that meetings be held in the hospital.

Section 3. The annual meeting shall be held in (month) of each year for the election and installation of officers, for receiving annual reports of officers, and for the conduct of such other business as may properly come before the meeting. Notice of the annual meeting shall be mailed to all members in good standing on the records of the auxiliary_____days in advance of said meeting.

Comment
> It is recommended that the annual meeting be held about a month after the end of the fiscal year. The fiscal year of the auxiliary should coincide with the fiscal year of the hospital. It is suggested that members be given adequate advance notice of the annual meeting, probably 30 days.

Section 4. _____per cent of the voting members shall constitute a quorum at any meeting of the auxiliary.

Comment
> The quorum should be stated as a percentage of the total membership. It should be kept low. Ordinarily, 10 or 15 per cent is an adequate percentage.

ARTICLE VI. OFFICERS

Section 1. The officers of the auxiliary shall be a president, a president-elect, a vice president for service, a vice president for community relations, a secretary, an assistant secretary, a treasurer, and an assistant treasurer. The president-elect shall serve in the absence of the president and shall assume the presidency should that office become vacant.

Comment

The above recommendation accomplishes several desirable results:

1. It provides for leadership training.
2. It provides for a president-elect, thus helping to secure continuity in the auxiliary's operations and giving the incumbent the incentive and time to prepare herself and her schedule for the job of president. At the same time, it provides for a presiding officer in the absence of the president and for an immediate successor should the president resign or become disabled during her term of office.
3. It avoids the danger, inherent in the traditional method of numbering vice presidents, that succession will be determined automatically by the numbers regardless of the leadership capabilities of the individuals occupying the vice presidential positions. At the same time, it gives each of the two vice presidents a general area of responsibility, paralleling the major functions of the auxiliary, and the opportunity to demonstrate their leadership potential.
4. It eases the executive burden that rests on the shoulders of the auxiliary president, while simultaneously providing better coordination among the organization's multiple activities.

Depending on their size, auxiliaries may need to adapt this pattern to fit their differing needs. A very small auxiliary may find that a president-elect and one additional vice president are adequate. A very large auxiliary may need both corresponding and recording secretaries (each with an assistant) and additional assistant treasurers.

Section 2. In the first year following the adoption of Article VI, "Officers," the auxiliary shall elect a president and a president-elect. Each shall serve one year only in her respective office. At the conclusion of that first year, the president-elect shall assume the office of president for one year only. Thereafter, the auxiliary shall elect each year a president-elect to serve for a period of one year, after which she shall automatically assume the office of president for one year. Persons who have held the office of president are then barred from reelection to the office of president-elect for a period of one year.

Model Bylaws/199

Comment

By limiting the tenure of office of the president and the president-elect to a period of one year, the possibility that the president-elect might not be reelected to a second term (along with the president), and therefore deprived of the presidency in the regular succession process, is eliminated. This provision also precludes the possibility that the president-elect will be serving for a total of four successive years (two years as president-elect and two years as president) in the auxiliary's most demanding jobs.

Section 3. All officers other than the president-elect shall be elected to serve for a term of one year and may be reelected for an additional term of one year in the same office. After election for two successive years to the same office, reelection to that office is barred for the period of one year.

Comment

Effort should be made to include in each year's slate of officers some who are new and some who are up for reelection.

Adequate leadership training should make it unnecessary to propose or elect to office a person who has already served two successive terms (two years) in that same office.

Section 4. The election of officers shall be held at the annual meeting. A slate of candidates shall be proposed by the nominating committee. Members eligible to vote may propose, from the floor, candidates for office.

Comment

A candidate's name should be proposed by the nominating committee or from the floor only with the candidate's express permission. Failure to secure the candidate's consent can cause embarrassment to the individual and problems for the auxiliary.

Section 5. The newly elected officers shall be installed at the annual meeting and take office immediately.

Comment

It is advisable that officers be elected and installed at the annual meeting to prevent any break in continuity between election and taking office, although the complete transfer of authority and records can only take place in the days following the annual meeting. A newly installed president will need time to appoint committee chairmen; outgoing officers and chairmen will need time to complete their records to turn over to their successors. However, the process should be accomplished as rapidly as possible.

Section 6. The unexpired term of any elected officer shall be filled by the board of directors after considering the recommendation of the nominating committee.

ARTICLE VII. DUTIES OF OFFICERS

Section 1. Duties of the president. As the chief executive officer of the auxiliary, the president shall serve as chairman of the auxiliary's board of directors and as the auxiliary's chief representative to the hospital and shall have supervision of the general management of the auxiliary. The president shall appoint, with the approval of the executive committee, the chairmen of all standing committees and the chairmen and members of such special committees as may be established, and shall be a member ex officio of all standing committees of the auxiliary. The president shall render a report on the activities of the auxiliary at least annually to the governing authority of the hospital and to the membership of the auxiliary and shall perform all other duties incident to the office of the president.

Comment

The provision that presidential appointees shall be made with the approval of the executive committee (that is, the elected members of the board) makes this a more democratic process by giving the membership a greater, though indirect, participation through all its elected representatives.

The term *standing committee* is defined in Article XI, Section 1.

Section 2. Duties of the president-elect. The president-elect shall, in the event of the absence, disability, or resignation of the president, assume the powers and perform the duties of the president. The president-elect shall be responsible for coordinating activities designed to maintain the organization and strengthen its capacity to serve and shall perform such other duties as may be delegated by the president or the board of directors of the auxiliary.

Section 3. Duties of the vice presidents. The vice president for service shall be responsible, subject to the direction of the president and the board of directors, for coordinating activities designed to implement the service function of the auxiliary. The vice president for community relations shall be responsible, subject to the direction of the president and the board of directors, for coordinating activities designed to implement the community relations function of the auxiliary.

In the event of the absence, disability, or resignation of the president and the president-elect, the vice president for service and the vice president for community relations shall, in that order, assume the powers and perform the duties of the president.

Section 4. Duties of the secretary. The secretary is the recording officer of the auxiliary and the custodian of its records, except such records that are specifically assigned to others. These records shall be open to the inspection of any member at all reasonable times. The secretary shall also be responsible for sending out notices of meetings of the auxiliary and for conducting the correspondence of the auxiliary except where otherwise provided.

Comment

Copies of the minutes of all auxiliary meetings should be filed with the hospital's governing authority as well as in the auxiliary's official files.

In some auxiliaries, the secretary's duties will be divided and the responsibility "for sending out notices of meetings of the auxiliary and for conducting the correspondence of the auxiliary" will be assigned to a corresponding secretary. The duties of the corresponding secretary, when such office exists, should be stipulated in a separate section of the bylaws.

Section 5. Duties of the assistant secretary. The assistant secretary shall assist the secretary and perform such duties as the secretary may delegate.

Comment

So that the assistant secretaryship may serve a useful training purpose, the person elected to the post should be assigned specific secretarial functions and responsibilities.

Section 6. Duties of the treasurer. The treasurer shall be responsible for keeping an accurate record of all financial affairs of the auxiliary, shall render an audited report to the hospital's governing authority and to the auxiliary at the end of the fiscal year, shall report to the annual meeting of the auxiliary, and shall render such interim reports as may be requested by the board of directors. The treasurer shall have charge of the auxiliary finances under the control and supervision of the board of direc-

tors and shall receive and expend all monies or funds of the
auxiliary in accordance with the provisions of Article XIII,
Sections 1 and 2.

Comment

The treasurer, and any others who handle monies for the
auxiliary, should be bonded at the expense of the auxiliary.
When there is bonding, the hospital's governing authority
makes the decision and determines the amount of the bonds.
Often the hospital bond can be extended to cover auxiliary
officers if the auxiliary is an integral part of the hospital
organization.

The treasurer's annual report should be audited by the
hospital's certified public accountant or another independent
auditor.

Section 7. Duties of the assistant treasurer. The assistant
treasurer shall assist the treasurer and perform such duties as
the treasurer may delegate.

Comment

Some auxiliaries may need more than one assistant treasurer.
However, regardless of the number, each assistant treasurer
should be assigned specific functions and responsibilities as
part of the assistant's training program.

ARTICLE VIII. BOARD OF DIRECTORS

Section 1. The board of directors of the auxiliary shall consist
of the officers of the auxiliary and the chairman of all standing
committees.

Comment

Board of directors here refers to the body having executive
powers within the auxiliary.

The most effective board is the so-called "working board,"
made up of persons who are on the board by virtue of their
positions as elected officers or appointed committee chairmen.
The working board has several advantages: its members are in
daily contact with the general membership; they are, as officers or chairmen, directly involved in the day-to-day activities
of the auxiliary and thus in a position to note trends, progress,
and problems, and to plan ahead.

Section 2. No director shall be eligible to serve more than
_____ successive years. After an absence from the board
of directors of at least one year, a member may be eligible for

election or appointment to a position that carries board membership.

Comment

Article VI, Section 2, limits the tenure of officers. The tenure of standing committee chairmen should also be limited, and the limit prescribed for the chairman of each committee should be included in the description of the committee set forth in the Administrative Policies and Procedures (see Article XI, Section 2). In addition, a board tenure provision is important to ensure frequent infusions of new blood into the auxiliary's executive body and to prevent the possibility of an uninterrupted exchange of chairs among officers and standing committee chairmen.

In determining the number of successive years a board member may serve, it is essential to strike a happy balance between the revitalizing effect of new members on the board and the demands of leadership development. Limiting a board member's tenure to six successive years would seem to strike the necessary balance, although some auxiliaries may, for good reason, decide to set a slightly higher limit.

A tenure provision avoids the danger of a static board. When the talents of potential leaders are used constructively during their prescribed one year's absence from the board, such a provision also gives new meaning to the concept of leadership development.

Section 3. All actions of the auxiliary's board of directors are subject to the approval of the governing board of the hospital or, if the governing authority so designates, to the approval of the hospital's chief executive officer. Within the above limitations, the board of directors shall be empowered to manage and control the property and funds of the auxiliary, to approve the auxiliary's annual operating budget, and to administer the affairs of the auxiliary on behalf of the auxiliary membership and in a manner consistent with these bylaws. Operating policies and procedures necessary to implement the basic policies set forth in the bylaws and to guide the operations of the auxiliary shall be recorded in the Administrative Policies and Procedures, a document that may be amended at any time by majority vote of the board of directors.

Comment

Section 3 may not be applicable where the auxiliary is a separate corporation or an unincorporated association.

The board's authority to approve the annual operating budget underscores its basic responsibility for establishing the auxiliary's program objectives and priorities for the coming year — an integral part of its overall planning responsibilities. A board-approved operating budget also becomes the treasurer's instrument of authorization for paying invoices on items covered in the budget.

When the auxiliary also has a financial contributions budget, as recommended in this manual, Section 3 must provide that the board of directors approve both budgets.

Section 4. The president shall report at each regular meeting of the auxiliary membership on auxiliary board actions taken subsequent to the last general meeting.

Section 5. Regular meetings of the board shall be held once a month, except as otherwise determined by the board, at such time and place as the board and/or the president may determine. Special meetings of the board may be held at any time and place determined by the president and, in addition, shall be called when requested in writing by not fewer than _____ of the members of the board. Directors shall be given not less than 48 hours' notice of special meetings. Notice may be waived if all directors sign a waiver, either before or after the special meeting.

The board of directors shall adopt its own rules for the conduct of its meetings not inconsistent with these bylaws.

Comment

The number of board members required to call a special meeting of the board should be stated as a percentage of the board's membership. The number needed should always be less than a majority, and one-fifth of the total board membership is the recommended number. Because the board meets frequently, it can be presumed that there must be a most urgent reason for a special meeting and, therefore, it should be possible for a relatively small group of the board to call such a meeting.

Section 6. _____ per cent of the members shall constitute a quorum at any meeting of the board. In the absence of a quorum, the meeting shall be adjourned.

Comment

The number of board members needed to constitute a quorum should be stated as a percentage of the board's total membership. Forty per cent is the recommended percentage figure.

Section 7. The board of directors shall be empowered to fill unexpired terms of officers and of elected members of the nominating committee occurring between annual meetings.

ARTICLE IX. EXECUTIVE COMMITTEE

Section 1. The executive committee shall consist of the president, the president-elect, the vice presidents, the secretary, and the treasurer.

Comment

Because even a working board may be a fairly large board (depending upon the number of standing committees the auxiliary has), it is well to provide for a small executive committee that can expedite matters when necessary. The executive committee is also useful as a planning group, a "president's cabinet." As such, it should meet regularly before each meeting of the board of directors to help the president plan the agenda, isolate any major problems facing the auxiliary, or consider long-range plans that will be presented later to the board. As an advisory group to the president, the executive committee can contribute to the smooth functioning of a very active auxiliary in which the president and the board carry a heavy work load. There are, however, dangers inherent in the use of the executive committee as a planning group, for it may become too authoritative and tend to undermine the power and prestige of the board.

An executive committee is not an essential functional element of an auxiliary. However, if an auxiliary is to have an executive committee, this committee must be provided for in the bylaws.

As elected officers of the auxiliary, the assistant secretary and the assistant treasurer sit on the auxiliary's board of directors, thus gaining valuable experience and training. However, to include them in the executive committee appears unnecessary in view of this committee's functions.

Section 2. The executive committee shall be empowered to act for the board of directors on all matters properly within the jurisdiction of the board, which the president determines cannot be held over until the next meeting of the board.

Section 3. All actions of the executive committee shall be reported to the board at its next meeting and shall be subject to revision and alteration by the board at such a meeting provided that no rights of third parties shall be adversely affected by such revision or alteration.

Section 4. Meetings of the executive committee may be held at any time and place determined by the president. Members of the executive committee shall be given not less than 12 hours' notice. Notice may be waived if all members sign a waiver either before or after the meeting.

ARTICLE X. NOMINATING COMMITTEE

Section 1. The nominating committee shall consist of a chairman and five members.

Comment

> The nominating committee functions throughout the year, seeking out leadership for the various positions to be filled and keeping appropriate records.

Section 2. The chairman of the nominating committee shall be the immediate past president of the auxiliary. If the immediate past president is unable or unwilling to serve, the president shall be authorized to appoint a chairman, with the approval of the executive committee.

Section 3. The president shall appoint, as one of the five members of the nominating committee, a member of the board of directors who shall be appointed to serve for a term of one year and shall be eligible for reappointment for one succeeding year. The remaining four members of the nominating committee shall be elected by the membership at the annual meeting. In the first year following the adoption of Article X, "Nominating Committee," the auxiliary shall elect two members to serve for two-year terms each and two members to serve for one-year terms each. Thereafter, two members shall be elected annually for terms of two years each.

Comment

> Several important principles underlie the composition of the nominating committee as suggested in these model bylaws.
> The provision that the immediate past president shall serve as chairman recognizes the value of her experience and her knowledge of the institution and offers her a post that is vital to the auxiliary's future programs. In making the immediate past president chairman of this committee, she is removed from current executive concerns, because these bylaws contain no

provision for the immediate past president to serve on the auxiliary's board of directors, and because the chairmanship of the nominating committee does not carry a seat on the board regardless of the individual filling it.

The nominating committee's need to be continually aware of current auxiliary activities, plans, and problems is ensured by the appointment of a member of the board of directors to the committee. Election by the general membership of the remaining four members of the committee on a rotating basis emphasizes the essential democratic nature of the auxiliary and ensures continuity, while simultaneously providing for a periodic infusion of new blood.

Section 4. Suggested nominations for officers of the auxiliary and for the elected members of the nominating committee shall be received by the nominating committee from the membership throughout the year and until_____days prior to the annual meeting. From these suggestions and as a result of its own deliberations, the nominating committee shall submit to the annual meeting a slate of candidates for offices and nominating committee membership for the ensuing year. This slate shall have been presented to the membership_____days prior to the annual meeting.

Membership on this committee does not preclude an individual's eligibility for nomination to an office within the auxiliary.

Section 5. The nominating committee shall submit for the consideration of the board of directors the names of persons to fill unexpired terms of officers and of elected members of the nominating committee occurring between annual meetings, when not otherwise provided for in the bylaws.

ARTICLE XI. STANDING COMMITTEES

Section 1. Standing committees include all regular committees of the auxiliary except the executive and nominating committees.

Comment

The executive and nominating committees are considered structural committees, specifically provided for in these bylaws.

Section 2. The standing committees of the auxiliary shall be authorized, created, and terminated by the board of directors according to the needs of the auxiliary. Each standing committee shall be named and described and its responsibilities delineated in the Administrative Policies and Procedures.

Comment

The number of standing committees will vary with each auxiliary, and they may be created or terminated as the occasion demands. Committees should be created only as there is a need for them; need will be determined by the size and functions of the individual auxiliary.

Section 3. The president shall appoint, with the approval of the executive committee, the chairmen of all standing committees. These chairmen, upon appointment by the president, become members of the board of directors.

Section 4. Each standing committee chairman, after conferring with the president, shall appoint members of her committee and shall designate one among them to serve as vice chairman.

Comment

The selection of committee members is a serious responsibility, because committee membership is the first step in leadership training. The position of vice chairman is especially important because, as a rule, future committee chairmen (and board members) are selected from among the individuals who have had experience as vice chairmen of committees. Each vice chairman should be selected with special care and should be given the opportunity to gain experience and develop her potential for leadership while in this office.

Section 5. The chairman of each standing committee shall file a summary report on the activities of the committee with the auxiliary secretary at least annually.

ARTICLE XII. AD HOC COMMITTEES

Section 1. Ad hoc committees may be authorized for specific tasks when need has been determined by the board of directors. At the time an ad hoc committee is established, the board shall specify the purpose and responsibilities of the committee, the number of individuals who will serve as members, and the specific types of expertise these individuals should possess.

Section 2. The president shall appoint, with the approval of the executive committee, the chairman and members of any ad hoc committee at the time of its authorization by the board.

Membership on an ad hoc committee need not be restricted to auxiliary members.

Comment

> Some auxiliaries may prefer that the chairman of an ad hoc committee have the prerogative of selecting committee members, in accordance with the guidelines established by the board for that committee. In this case, Section 2 of Article XII would be changed to reflect this decision.

Section 3. An ad hoc committee shall be terminated automatically when its assigned task is completed or at the direction of the board of directors.

ARTICLE XIII. FINANCES

Section 1. All monies or funds received or expended by the auxiliary shall be duly entered in the treasurer's books.

Section 2. All expenditures, other than those authorized in the annual operating budget, must be approved by the board of directors. Expenditure of proceeds from all fund-raising activities of the auxiliary shall further be subject to the approval of the hospital governing authority.

Section 3. All contracts made, accepted, or executed by the auxiliary shall be signed by the president or her authorized representative and countersigned by an appropriate official of the hospital.

Comment

> Section 3 is not applicable to a separately incorporated auxiliary or an unincorporated association.

Section 4. All bank accounts of the auxiliary shall be established by resolution of the hospital's governing authority.

Comment

> The provision set forth in Section 4 is important as evidence of the fact that the auxiliary operates as an integral part of the hospital. This provision is not applicable if the auxiliary is separately incorporated or an unincorporated association.

Section 5. All checks drawn against funds of the auxiliary shall be signed by the treasurer. In the absence of the treasurer, checks shall be signed by the assistant treasurer.

Comment

In view of the restrictions placed upon the expenditure of auxiliary funds by the provisions of Section 2 of this article, it would seem unnecessary to require any countersignature on auxiliary checks.

Comment

Depending on local law, the attorney consulted may make a number of suggestions differing from the model bylaws or these comments. Article XIII is particularly susceptible to attorney-recommended variations. The attorney's suggestions as to this article may include particular provisions to ensure compliance with conditions of federal income tax exemption of the auxiliary or the institution itself.

With reference to Article XIII, an auxiliary often must include, as a separate section of this article, legal provision for the disposal of funds and assets in the event that the auxiliary is dissolved or its institution closes or changes ownership.

For an auxiliary that is organized as an integral part of its institution, or as an unincorporated association, any remaining funds at the time of dissolution should be given to the institution, and this directive should be clearly stated in the auxiliary's bylaws.

Regarding a separately incorporated auxiliary, most states require that a provision for dissolution and subsequent disposition of funds be made in the group's charter when it files its original articles of incorporation. The charter should state that remaining funds be given to the institution. In states where this legal requirement is not present, the provision should be incorporated into the auxiliary's bylaws.

In the event that the institution dissolves, the auxiliary's bylaws can state that the auxiliary's funds be given to a successor hospital or another charitable institution in the area.

If the institution is a voluntary, not-for-profit hospital, and it is purchased by an investor-owned hospital corporation, then the tax status of the auxiliary would change. Before the transaction is completed the auxiliary's board can take any action necessary to provide for the contingency.

ARTICLE XIV. FISCAL YEAR

The fiscal year shall commence_____and shall end_____.

Comment

The auxiliary's fiscal year should coincide with the fiscal year of the hospital.

ARTICLE XV. PARLIAMENTARY AUTHORITY

Parliamentary authority for the hospital auxiliary shall be *Robert's Rules of Order, Newly Revised* (Glenview, Ill.: Scott, Foresman and Co.), 1970 (ref. 49).

ARTICLE XVI. AMENDMENTS

These bylaws may be altered, repealed, or amended by the affirmative vote of two-thirds of the members present and voting at any regular or special meeting of the auxiliary, provided that notice of the proposed alteration, repeal, or amendment is contained in the notice of such meeting, which has been mailed not less than 14 days in advance of the meeting. No amendment to the bylaws shall become effective until approved by the governing authority of (name of institution).

ARTICLE XVII. APPROVAL AND ADOPTION

These bylaws, upon approval of the hospital's governing authority, shall be effective immediately on affirmative vote of two-thirds of the auxiliary members present and voting.

Approved by Board of Trustees of (name of institution)

Date_____

President of Board of Trustees_____

Secretary_____

Adopted by (name of auxiliary)   Date_____

President_____

Secretary_____

Comment

Apart from other considerations, the governing authority's approval of auxiliary bylaws is required by the current standards of the Joint Committee on Accreditation of Hospitals.

appendix B
Sample Provision in Hospital Corporation Bylaws to Establish or Recognize a Volunteer Organization

ARTICLE 00
VOLUNTEER ORGANIZATION

Section 1. The governing board is authorized to designate a volunteer organization (auxiliary) for the hospital and to provide for its organization as an integral part of the hospital corporation.

Section 2. The designated organization may perform patient-related services within or outside of the hospital, conduct fund-raising activities, conduct community service projects, enter into contracts as approved by the hospital administrator, and carry on such other activities necessary to accomplish its purposes as approved by the governing board.

Section 3. The designated organization may establish bank accounts. Any such accounts opened must be authorized by the governing board. The hospital treasurer may delegate to elected officers of the volunteer organization (auxiliary) the authority to disburse funds on behalf of the organization. Funds disbursed for

By whatever form the governing body determines to establish, recognize, or affiliate with a volunteer organization (auxiliary), legal counsel of the governing body should be consulted. The above is an example of establishment or recognition being conferred by a bylaws provision of the hospital corporation. Legal counsel may suggest another form, such as a board resolution, and different or additional terms appropriate to the individual situation.

the benefit of the hospital must have the prior approval of the administrator.

Section 4. The designated organization shall file annually with the governing board an audited financial statement, a report of the orgonization's activities during the past year, and a report of proposed activities for the coming year. The reports must be filed within 60 days of the close of the designated organization's fiscal year.

appendix C
The American Hospital Association As a Resource

A health care institution's membership in the American Hospital Association automatically includes services to the auxiliary associated with that institution. As a resource for definitive information on the health care field in general, and for specific guidelines to the functioning of auxiliaries, the Association can furnish a broad spectrum of services to the auxiliary wishing to increase its effectiveness.

Such services can be obtained through utilization of the following sources of assistance:

- AHA publications
- The AHA library
- Meetings that provide educational opportunities
- Consultation furnished by AHA staff

AHA Publications

Periodicals

On a regular basis, auxiliaries receive several periodicals, including *The Volunteer Leader,* a journal devoted to the concerns and interests of auxilians and directors of volunteer services; *Washington Developments,* a review of health care legislation, which is published by the AHA's Washington office; and *Hospital Week,* a capsule summary of news of interest to health care institutions.

Special note should be made here of how AHA material sent to auxiliaries is addressed. All material intended for the use of the auxiliary is sent to the attention of the auxiliary president, in care of the institution. Mail is addressed this way, rather than to individual auxiliary presidents by name and home address, because presidents change frequently — many yearly — and it is costly and impractical to maintain a list of some 4,000 individuals and their home addresses. The auxiliary president is responsible for making whatever local arrangements are necessary to ensure that she receives the AHA mail addressed to her attention.

Auxilians should also read the AHA periodical *Hospitals, Journal of the American Hospital Association,* which is published bimonthly and distributed to the chief executives of health care institutions; it is available to others by subscription.

Of course, *all* AHA periodicals can be obtained by subscription. The auxiliary's leadership should take advantage of this fact and ensure that such publications are made available to board members and general membership alike. If this means taking out several subscriptions to *The Volunteer Leader,* for example, then provision should be made within the auxiliary's budget for these subscriptions, and they should be designated as an expense of membership education.

Catalogs

Auxiliaries also receive the AHA *Publications Catalog,* which is published annually, and the *Film Catalog,* which is published periodically. Additional single copies of both catalogs are available from the Association free upon request.

The *Publications Catalog* lists manuals, brochures, pamphlets, and reference materials, many of which are relevant to auxiliaries. Also included are listings of tapes, posters, and packaged educational programs. The *Film Catalog* offers an alphabetical list of films and filmstrips available from the American Hospital Association and other distributors, describing content and stating rental or purchase price. Rental or purchase arrangements can be made by contacting the Association's Film Library.

Other Publications

When the Association publishes a new manual, brochure, pamphlet, or other material that has application to or interest for auxiliaries, a copy is automatically sent to each auxiliary.

Library Services

The Library of the American Hospital Association, Asa S. Bacon Memorial, contains one of the largest collections of hospital literature in the world. Of its many services provided to member institutions and therefore to their auxiliaries, the loan service is probably the most useful in terms of the auxiliary's needs. Auxilians can borrow a collection of literature — books, articles, and pamphlets — on any subject related to health care administration. Materials specifically related to the interests of auxiliaries comprise a significant part of the library's total collection.

A loan made to an individual consists of a *representative* collection of published material rather than a comprehensive one. In other words, materials supplied on a specific subject do not include every article, book, or brochure on that subject, but rather a selection from what is available.

Borrowing can be done by personal visit to the library, by mail, or by phone. A request for information should be as clear and specific as possible, briefly describing the purpose for which the material will be used and delimiting the subject. It would be inappropriate, for example, for an auxilian to request "all the information available on auxiliaries." This is far too broad and would require a much too comprehensive collection of material. Rather, the request should be along the lines of specific subjects, such as membership recruitment, organizing a new auxiliary, legal aspects of the auxiliary's operations, fund raising, and so forth. If the individual requesting material *does* need to know "everything" about auxiliaries, then this manual, which can be purchased from the Association, would be an appropriate reference.

When requests for information include references to specific publications, such references should be as accurate, complete, and detailed as possible, providing, when known, the author, title, and publisher of books and the author, title of article, title of journal, volume, page number, and date of journal articles. The period of the loan varies from two weeks to one month, depending upon the current popularity of the subject matter requested and the amount of available literature on the subject maintained by the library. Generally, an individual can obtain a month's renewal of material if requested. The only cost for borrowing publications is the postage required when returning materials by mail. There is no charge for lending materials by mail or for in-person transactions.

For auxilians wishing to obtain a comprehensive list of references on every aspect of hospital administration, in order to obtain background information in the field, the *Hospital Literature Index* is available. This compilation, published quarterly, lists articles, by subject and author, for more than 500 journals. The last issue of the year is an annual cumulation. Every five years, the information is combined into the *Cumulative Index of Hospital Literature*. Auxilians should check their institutions' libraries for availability of this publication.

Educational Opportunities

The American Hospital Association offers a variety of institutes, seminars, workshops, and conferences on significant subject matter, some designed specifically for auxilians and others furnishing information to which auxilians can relate. The meetings for auxilians, which are coordinated by the Association's Division of Volunteer Services, focus primarily on providing techniques for the effective management of the auxiliary in all aspects of its operations.

Information concerning subject, content, date, and location of such meetings is published in *Hospitals, J.A.H.A.*, and *The Volunteer Leader*. Prior to these events, announcements are also sent out to auxiliaries, addressed to the attention of the president.

The American Hospital Association's annual convention, held in the late summer, devotes a portion of its program to the concerns and interests of auxilians. It also offers a broader range of subject matter about the health care field, to which auxilians can relate.

Another educational opportunity is the AHA annual meeting in Washington, D.C., when auxilians can learn of the Association's positions on various matters of health care legislation, followed by their personal participation in the legislative process.

In addition to a business session of the AHA House of Delegates, the Association conducts a special briefing on its legislative viewpoint pertaining to health care, thus preparing participants for meetings with their representatives in Congress. These meetings offer those attending the opportunity to exchange opinions with legislators on the various issues affecting the health care field and hospitals and enable auxilians to have actual input into legislative activity on behalf of health care.

Consultation Services

Auxiliaries requiring individual assistance in resolving problems, in strengthening their organizations for more effective functioning, or in planning special educational programs at the state or local levels can look to the American Hospital Association for help. Various divisions within the Association can be of aid to auxiliaries, meeting specific problems with specific expertise. However, it is the Division of Volunteer Services that is particularly attuned to the interests of auxiliaries and qualified to offer the kind of comprehensive consultation services that auxiliaries may require. These services to membership are always available by mail, telephone, or personal visits to AHA headquarters in Chicago. In addition, on-site visits, at the request of the auxiliary and its institution, can be arranged.

To obtain further information, auxiliaries should contact the Division of Volunteer Services of the American Hospital Association, 840 North Lake Shore Drive, Chicago, Ill. 60611, telephone (312) 645-9400.

appendix D
Statement on the
Role of the Auxiliary
on the Health Care Team

Preamble

The accessibility, the acceptability, and the costs of health care are matters of great public concern today, and the public is turning to hospitals, as the major health resources in their communities, for answers. Hospitals, for their part, recognize that finding acceptable answers requires broad community participation in defining the problems and broad community support in achieving the solutions.

Auxilians are citizen volunteers who, having a common commitment to the goals of their hospitals and a common concern for the health of their communities, have joined forces in collective efforts to assist hospitals in the delivery of health care.

Throughout the years, auxiliaries have been many things to their hospitals. They have been sources of financial assistance and of volunteer manpower. They have served as persuasive voices for hospitals in their communities. Whatever the needs of their hospitals, auxiliaries have responded — and in their response have demonstrated the value of hospital-affiliated voluntary community organizations through which the multiple talents of the concerned community can be deployed.

Having proved their flexibility and their diverse capabilities in the past, auxiliaries are a logical source of assistance in meeting the present needs of their hospitals. As established channels

Approved by the American Hospital Association, May 6-8, 1970.

for community participation in hospital affairs, they provide a base on which to build an expanded hospital-community relationship.

Auxiliaries have a new opportunity for service today, and hospitals seeking to interrelate more effectively with their communities have a ready source of aid. How well auxiliaries will respond depends on their ability to broaden the base of community participation in their own organizations and activities. How well hospitals will utilize this source of aid depends on a reassessment of the appropriate role of auxiliaries on the health care team.

The American Hospital Association offers the following six-point statement as a guide to each member hospital in reexamining the role of its auxiliary in the light of today's needs for community involvement and support.

The Role of the Auxiliary on the Health Care Team

1. The auxiliary is an integral part of the institutional organization: self-governing but nonautonomous; exercising certain rights, as authorized by the hospital's governing body, to represent and assist the institution; and responsible in the exercise of these rights to administration. By virtue of its place within the total organization, there is a direct line of communication between administration and the auxiliary's leadership.

2. Changes taking place in hospitals in response to technological and societal changes affect all parts of the organization, including the auxiliary. In consequence, the long-standing definition of auxiliary purpose has been expanded to read "to render service to_____Hospital and its patients and to assist_____Hospital in promoting the health and welfare of the community in accordance with objectives established by the hospital." If this augmented purpose is to be fulfilled, an auxiliary must be acutely aware of social changes in its community and persistent in its efforts to find effective means of assisting its own and related agencies in the delivery of optimum health care to all community members.

3. Administration regards the auxiliary in two lights: (a) as a trusted member of the institution's team, which can mean

involving the auxiliary's leadership in discussion of the institution's long-range plans, or taking leadership into its confidence on current issues (such as hospital costs and rates) ; and (b) as a community resource, to be consulted in determining community attitudes and with capabilities of initiating and carrying out community-oriented projects.

4. The auxiliary recognizes that it is a part of the institutional organization and understands that it must work within the framework of its institutional relationship. At the same time, it is seeking a role that is relevant to the current and future needs of its institution and its community, and one that utilizes to the fullest extent its capabilities as a voluntary community organization to aid in improving the delivery of health care.

5. The auxiliary continues to be a valued source of support and recruitment for the institution's inservice volunteer program. However, to equate the auxiliary solely with that program, or to consider it as an appendage of the volunteer services department, is to take a shortsighted view of the auxiliary's total capabilities.

   As the auxiliary's concept of "hospital service" enlarges to encompass service to the community as well as service to patients and to the hospital, and as its activities become more diverse, its network of departmental relationships within the hospital grows correspondingly. Through appropriate committees and with the approval of administration, the auxiliary cooperates with the public relations department, the development department, and possibly others in much the same way as it has traditionally cooperated with the volunteer services department.

6. Funds raised by the auxiliary are important to the institution's capital needs, and to support institutional and community health programs for which outside financing may be unavailable. The auxiliary selects a method of fund raising that: (a) best reflects the image the institution wishes to project, (b) complements the auxiliary's own service and community relations functions, and (c) is most acceptable to the community. These goals may be achieved by service-oriented projects and by auxiliary fund-raising activities undertaken as part of the institution's overall fund-raising

effort. However, an overemphasis on fund raising can undermine these goals, and may deter the recruitment of new members.

References

In the development of this manual, numerous sources of information were used. These references are listed below.

1. American Hospital Association. *Auxiliary Gift and Coffee Shop Management.* Chicago: AHA, 1962.
2. _____. *Blood Project File: Guidelines for Auxiliary Programs Supporting the Voluntary Donation and Replacement of Blood.* Chicago: AHA, 1969.
3. _____. *Financial Aid Programs in Support of Health Occupations: A Guide for Auxiliaries.* Chicago: AHA, 1971.
4. _____. *Guidelines for Auxiliary Fund Raising.* Chicago: AHA, 1965.
5. _____. *Guidelines to Federal Legislative Action for Auxilians.* Chicago: AHA, 1973.
6. _____. *Patterns and Principles for Hospital Auxiliaries.* Chicago: AHA, 1957 (out of print).
7. _____. *Planning Educational Programs for Hospital Auxiliaries.* Chicago: AHA, 1955.
8. _____. *The Practice of Planning in Health Care Institutions.* Chicago: AHA, 1973.
9. _____. *Statement on Optimum Health Services.* Chicago: AHA, 1965.
10. _____. *Volunteer Recognition and Identification.* Chicago: AHA, 1967.
11. _____. *The Volunteer Services Department in a Health Care Institution.* Chicago: AHA, 1973.
12. _____. *What Is Your Auxiliary's H.I.Q. (Hospital Information Quotient)?* Chicago: AHA, 1962 (out of print).
13. American Society for Hospital Public Relations of the American Hospital Association. *A Basic Guide to Hospital Public Relations.* Chicago: AHA, 1973.
14. Balfanz, D. Chat with the chairman. *The Auxiliary Leader.* 8:6, Jan. 1967.

15. _____. Chat with the chairman. *The Auxiliary Leader.* 8:5, Apr. 1967.
16. _____. How effective is your auxiliary? *The Auxiliary Leader.* 2:13, Oct. 1961.
17. Buchanan, R. D., and Schmidt, W. I. Effective staff meetings. *Cornell Hotel and Restaurant Association Quarterly.* 12:104, May 1971.
18. Clark, N. F. Relating auxiliary meetings to the auxiliary's purpose. *The Auxiliary Leader.* 5:8, Dec. 1964.
19. Cooper, S. S. Committees that work. *Journal of Nursing Administration.* 3:30, Jan.-Feb. 1973.
20. Counihan, D. M. The proper handling of an association meeting. *American Society of Association Executives' Journal.* 13:56, Oct. 1961.
21. Danielson, J. M. The importance of planning. *The Auxiliary Leader.* 1:14, Nov. 1960.
22. Decker, Mrs. T. Auxiliary programming bridges hospital-public communications gap. *The Volunteer Leader.* 12:1, June 1971.
23. Duda, S. Inservice training of volunteers. Speech presented at 1973 American Health Congress, Chicago.
24. Educate yourselves first, then patients, auxilians are · told. *The Volunteer Leader.* 13:15, May 1972.
25. Evaluation: a forum for human service decision-makers. *Evaluation.* 1:2, Fall 1972.
26. Flanders, C. Auxiliaries now and in the future—action-planning in a period of change. Part 1. *The Auxiliary Leader.* 8:1, July 1967.

27. _____. Auxiliaries now and in the future—action-planning in a period of change. Part 2. *The Auxiliary Leader.* 8:6, Aug. 1967.
28. Gordon, A., and Gordon, A. *Techniques of Successful Fund Raising: A Handbook.* New York: Exposition Press, 1967.
29. Gower, Mrs. S. M. The measure of an auxiliary: its commitment to improved health care. *The Volunteer Leader.* 13:1, Jan. 1972.
30. The Hospital Association of Pennsylvania and the Pennsylvania Association of Hospital Auxiliaries. *Hospital Auxiliary Handbook.* Camp Hill, Pa.: HAP and PAHA, 1971.
31. Knappenberger, Mrs. H. D. Making the most of auxiliary meeting programs. *The Volunteer Leader.* 12:9, May 1971.
32. Koestler, F. A. *Creative Annual Reports.* New York: National Public Relations Council of Health and Welfare Services, Inc., 1969.
33. Levey, S., and Loomba, N. P. *Health Care Administration: A Managerial Perspective.* Philadelphia: J. B. Lippincott Co., 1973.
34. Millham, Mrs. N. Chat with the chairman. *The Auxiliary Leader.* 9:7, Jan. 1968.
35. _____. Chat with the chairman. *The Volunteer Leader.* 10:6, Mar. 1969.
36. _____. Components of effective program planning. *The Volunteer Leader.* 10:3, June 1969.
37. _____. Let's put meaning into our meetings. *The Auxiliary Leader.* 6:1, Feb. 1965.

38. _____. New services help auxiliary meet its expanded responsibilities. *The Volunteer Leader.* 13:1, June 1972.

39. _____. Speech presented at annual meeting of West Virginia Association of Hospital Auxiliaries, Oct. 19, 1971.

40. Milton, Mrs. H. Auxiliary organizational structure: good records are the key to sound management. *The Auxiliary Leader.* 4:13, Mar. 1963.

41. National Center for Voluntary Action. Materials on volunteer recruitment and fund raising. Washington, D.C.: NCVA, 1972-73.

42. National Center for Voluntary Action. Midwest Regional Conference, Sept. 14-16, 1972. Discussion on fund raising.

43. *Officers' Guide for Twig Groups.* Dayton, Ohio: The Children's Medical Center, 1973.

44. O'Neill, Mrs. J. F. Planning for program and evaluating progress. Speech presented at Seminar on Leadership, Hospital Association of New York State, Syracuse, Jan. 1967.

45. Piraino, T. A. On the minutes of the meeting. *The Office.* 66:12, July 1967.

46. Prince, G. M. How to be a better meeting chairman. *Harvard Business Review.* 47:98, Jan.-Feb. 1969.

47. Questions and answers. *The Volunteer Leader.* 13:20, June 1972.

48. Risley, M. *House of Healing: The Story of the Hospital.* Garden City, N.Y.: Doubleday, 1961.

49. Robert, H. M. *Robert's Rules of Order, Newly Revised.* Glenview, Ill.: Scott, Foresman and Co., 1970.

50. Salasin, S. What is evaluation good for? *Evaluation.* 1:2, Fall 1972.

51. Saltsman, Mrs. J. A. Chat with the chairman. *The Volunteer Leader.* 12:6, Sept. 1971.

52. _____. Chat with the chairman. *The Volunteer Leader.* 13:13, Sept. 1972.

53. Shepperd, J. B. *The President's Guide to Club and Organization Management and Meetings.* New York City: Hawthorn Books, Inc., 1961.

54. Staff meetings and conferences. *Administrative Briefs.* 11:1, Apr. 1968.

55. Strauss, B., and Strauss, F. *New Ways to Better Meetings.* New York City: Viking Press, 1964.

56. Sussmann, P. Presentation at Conference on Future of Auxilians, Mar. 2-3, 1970, American Hospital Association, Chicago.

57. Swift, H., and Swift, E. *Community Groups and You.* New York City: John Day Company, 1964.

58. Turner, Mrs. H. A. Does auxiliary fund use reflect community need? *The Volunteer Leader.* 11:1, Aug. 1970.

59. Two cases demonstrate a natural evolution: hospital consolidations lead to shared auxiliary services. *The Volunteer Leader.* 14:8, June 1973.

60. United Hospital Fund of New York. *Essentials for Hospital Auxiliaries — A Guide.* New York City: UHFNY, 1963.

61. U.S. Department of Health, Education, and Welfare. *Guidelines for Health Services Research and Development: Shared Services* (DHEW Pub. [HSM] 72-3023). Washington, D.C.: U.S. Government Printing Office, Feb. 1972.

62. Webster, E. Another meeting. *Management Review.* 51:4, Oct. 1962.

63. Wilbraham, A. L. Evaluation: an essential component of the leadership process. *The Volunteer Leader.* 11:7, Sept. 1970.

64. Wilsey, Mrs. H. L. Evaluation: key to identifying the reasons for successes and failures. *The Volunteer Leader.* 11:10, July 1970.

65. _____. How does the auxiliary fit into long-range planning? *The Volunteer Leader.* 11:1, Jan. 1970.

Index

V

312972